CARDIOVASCULAR–RENAL
Axis Disorders
in Dogs and Cats

Plaza Antonio Beltrán Martínez nº 1, planta 8 - letra I
(Centro empresarial El Trovador)
50002 Zaragoza - Spain

First printing: January 2021

This book was originally published in Spanish under the title:
Alteraciones del eje cardiovascular-renal en el perro y en el gato
© 2019 Grupo Asís Biomedia, SL
ISBN Spanish edition: 978-84-17640-72-9

Translation:
Ubiqus

Illustrator:
Jacob Gragera Artal

ISBN: 978-84-18020-55-1
DL: Z 1692-2020

Design, layout and printing:
Grupo Asís Biomedia, SL
www.grupoasis.com
info@grupoasis.com

GRUPO asis

edra is an imprint of Grupo Asís

Warning:

Veterinary science is constantly evolving, as are pharmacology and the other sciences. Inevitably, it is therefore the responsibility of the veterinary surgeon to determine and verify the dosage, the method of administration, the duration of treatment and any possible contraindications to the treatments given to each individual patient, based on his or her professional experience. Neither the publisher nor the author can be held liable for any damage or harm caused to people, animals or properties resulting from the correct or incorrect application of the information contained in this book.

CARDIOVASCULAR RENAL
Axis Disorders
in Cats and Dogs

Javier Duque Carrasco
Rafael Barrera Chacón
Alicia Caro Vadillo
M.ª Ángeles Daza González
Gonzalo Marcos Gómez
M.ª Victoria Mogollón Jiménez
David Chipayo Gonzales
Domingo Casamián Sorrosal
Fernando Martínez Taboada

edra

Wherever you are – I am sure smiling proudly and always convinced that it was worthwhile – this book is for you, mother. And because you, Celia, were there at my side, it is for you, too. Thank you for respecting the times and bearing the absences. Thank you for making room in your big heart, where thousand works like this one would fit.

Javier Duque

To my wife, Isabel, and my children, Rafael and Gonzalo.

Rafael Barrera

To Elena and Julia for making Berlingtonia exist. To my mentors Sonja Fonfara, Sheena Warman and Kate Murphy. To Javier and Rafa, for inviting me to collaborate on this book. To my parents.

Domingo Casamián

To Nicola and my children, Rafa and Santi. Every hour dedicated to any of my projects is an hour away from you. Thank you for your understanding.

Fernando Martínez

THE AUTHORS

Javier Duque Carrasco

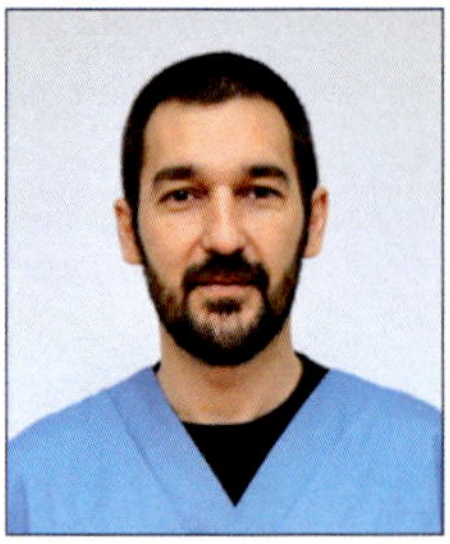

Degree in veterinary medicine from the University of Extremadura (UEx) in 2000 and PhD from the same university in 2013. He first worked as a veterinary surgeon in a private clinic (2000–2005) and later joined the Internal Medicine Service at the UEx Veterinary Teaching Hospital. He is currently a professor in the Animal Medicine Department at the Faculty of Veterinary Medicine of Cáceres (UEx).

He has furthered his training at the hospitals of the faculties of Bristol, Liverpool (United Kingdom) and North Carolina (United States) and at the Virgen del Rocío (Seville) and San Pedro de Alcántara (Cáceres) human medicine hospitals. He is a member of the European Society of Veterinary Cardiology (ESVC). He has published articles in several national and international journals.

Rafael Barrera Chacón

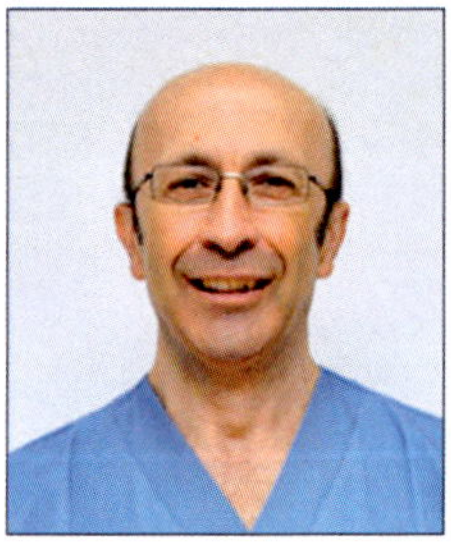

Degree in veterinary medicine from the University of Córdoba in 1984 and PhD from the University of Extremadura (UEx) in 1989. He is a lecturer in the Animal Medicine Department of the UEx, director of the UEx Veterinary Teaching Hospital, and head of his clinical pathology laboratory.

He was a visiting fellow at several universities such as the National Veterinary School of Alfort (France), the National Autonomous University of Mexico (UNAM) and the University of Chile. He is the author of several publications in Spanish and international journals and has given lectures on clinical pathology both in Spain and abroad. He is currently working on the characterisation of biomarkers of renal disease in dogs.

Alicia Caro Vadillo

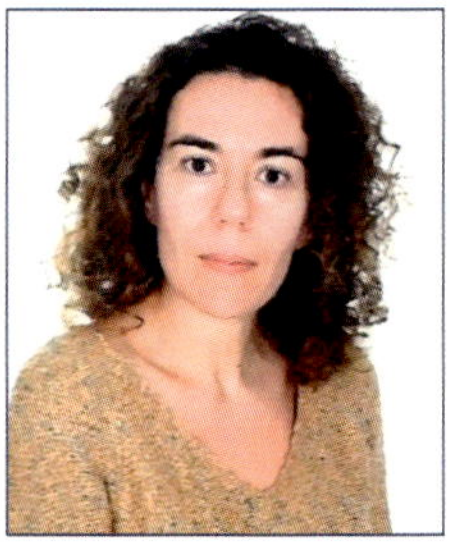

She graduated in veterinary medicine in 1994 and earned her PhD in veterinary medicine in 1999 from the Complutense University of Madrid (UCM). She furthered her training in small animal internal medicine at the University of California-Davis (United States) (1996) and at human medicine university hospitals (San Carlos University Teaching Hospital) (2002). She is a lecturer in the Department of Animal Medicine and Surgery of the Faculty of Veterinary Medicine of the UCM, member of the

Small Animal Internal Medicine Service at the UCM Veterinary Teaching Hospital and head of the Cardiology and Respiratory Diseases Unit of this service.

She is a certified member of the Working Group on Cardiology and Respiratory Diseases of AVEPA. She has published more than 50 articles in Spanish and international journals and has collaborated in the preparation of book chapters and monographs on heart disease and respiratory disease in small animals. She is the director of the UCM Diploma Course on Heart Disease in Small Animals.

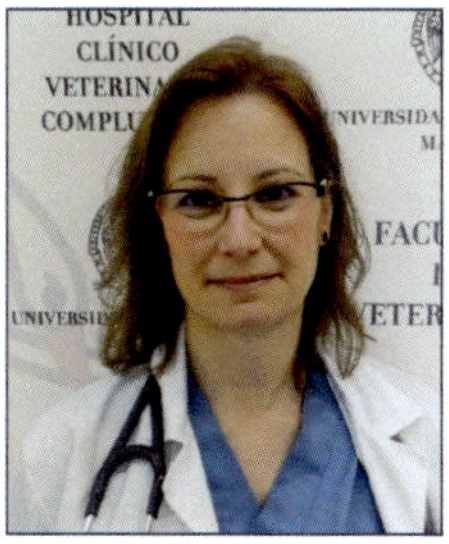

M.ª Ángeles Daza González

She graduated in veterinary medicine in 1998 and obtained a PhD in veterinary medicine in 2016 from the Complutense University of Madrid (UCM). She is AVEPA-certified in emergency and intensive care. She has worked at the Experimental Unit of La Paz University Hospital in Madrid and the Emergency and Intensive Care Unit of the University of North Carolina (United States).

Since 2006 she has worked as a full-time veterinary surgeon in the Hospitalisation and Intensive Care Service and is head of the Nephrology and Urology Unit of the Small Animal Medicine Service at the UCM Veterinary Teaching Hospital.

She is a member of the European Veterinary Emergency and Critical Care Society (EVECCS) and Veterinary Emergency and Critical Care Society (VECCS). She has published several articles and has been a speaker at emergency and intensive care congresses.

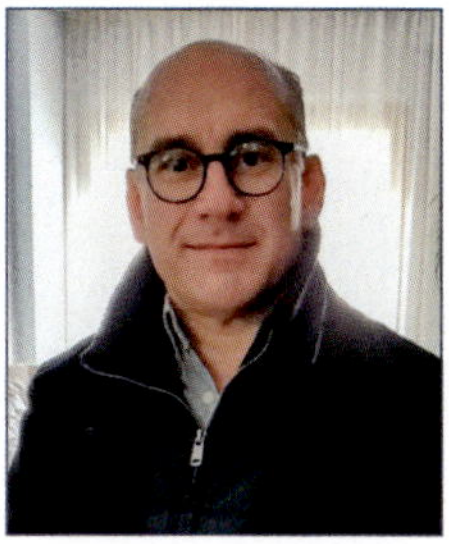

Gonzalo Marcos Gómez

He graduated in medicine from the University of Extremadura in 1987, and completed his residency in cardiology at the Institute of Cardiology of Madrid from 1989 to 1993. He then completed several postgraduate training programmes, including a postgraduate diploma as part of the Programme for Leadership and Management of Clinical Cardiology Units (ESADE-SEC-Ferrer), a Master's Degree in Cardiology from the University of Elche-SEC-Menarini (2011), a Master's Degree in Clinical Unit Management from the University of Murcia-IMAS (2015–2016) and a postgraduate programme in acute heart failure from the Francisco de Vitoria University (2016).

From 2007 to 2013 he was head of the Cardiology Service at the Hospital San Pedro de Alcántara of Cáceres and since 2013 he has been the director of the Cardiac Imaging Unit.

He has participated in several medical trials, collaborated on a number of international publications and communications for both Spanish and international congresses, and has been a speaker at Spanish and international congresses.

M.ª Victoria Mogollón Jiménez

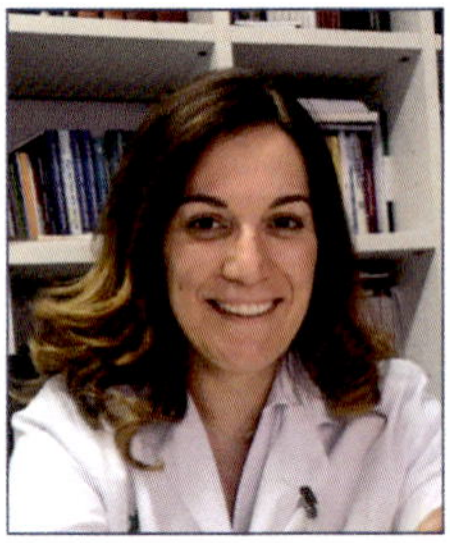

She graduated in medicine from the University of León in 2002. She obtained her diploma as a cardiology specialist at the Virgen del Rocío University Hospital (Seville) in 2008. She completed a PhD Programme in Biomedical Research (University of Seville) in 2008. Certified in Adult Transthoracic Echocardiography by the European Society of Cardiology in 2009. Master's Degree in Cardiology in 2012 and Master's Degree in Diagnostic Imaging in 2014 from Miguel Hernández University of Elche. Master's Degree in Acute Heart Care from the Catholic University of Murcia in 2015. International Master's Degree in Pulmonary Hypertension from the International University Menéndez Pelayo in 2016.

She has served as a cardiologist, initially at the Hospital of Mérida and subsequently at the San Pedro de Alcántara University Hospital of Cáceres. She currently divides her healthcare activity between two main areas: she is part of the Heart Imaging Unit and head of the Hereditary Heart Disease Unit of the San Pedro de Alcántara University Hospital of Cáceres.

She has written several articles published in books in Spanish and in both Spanish and international publications, and has participated in several clinical trials.

David Chipayo Gonzales

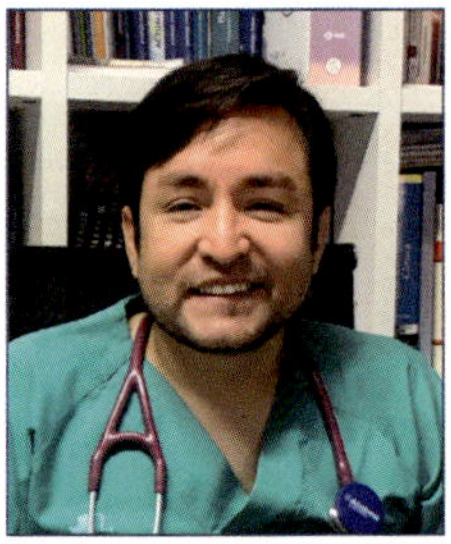

Degree in medicine by the University of San Martín de Porres of Lima (Peru) in 2009. Residency in nephrology at Dos de Mayo National Hospital of Lima (Peru) from 2011 to 2014.

He is currently a resident in cardiology at the San Pedro de Alcántara University Hospital of Cáceres.

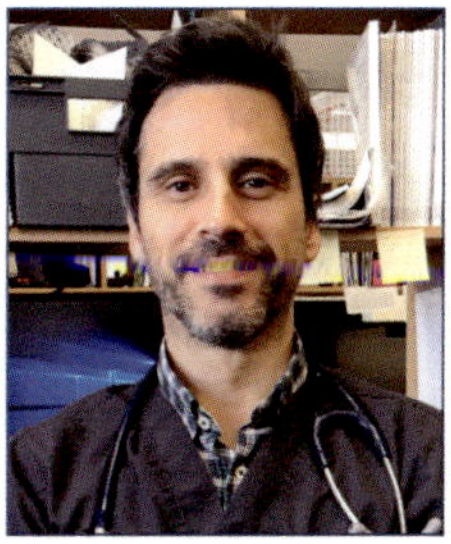

Domingo Casamián Sorrosal

Degree in veterinary medicine from the University of Zaragoza. He completed a general internship at the Animal Medical Centre in Manchester and worked at several hospitals in the United Kingdom, during which time he became an Royal College Veterinary Surgeons (RCVS) specialist in small animal internal medicine and veterinary cardiology. He completed a residency in small animal internal medicine (3 years) and in veterinary cardiology (4 years) at the University of Bristol Referral Hospital, after which earned a European specialist diploma in internal medicine and the British specialist diploma in veterinary cardiology. He remained at the University of Bristol first as a clinician and then as the head of the Cardiorespiratory Service until July 2016. He is currently head of the Cardiology and Cardiopulmonary Medicine Service at Southfields Veterinary Specialists, a referral hospital in Basildon (United Kingdom) and professor at the Catholic University of Valencia. He also works as a cardiology and respiratory specialist at the university's Veterinary Teaching Hospital.

He has published numerous articles in scientific journals in his field, has written book chapters, has been a speaker at Spanish and international congresses and is a reviewer in various veterinary scientific journals.

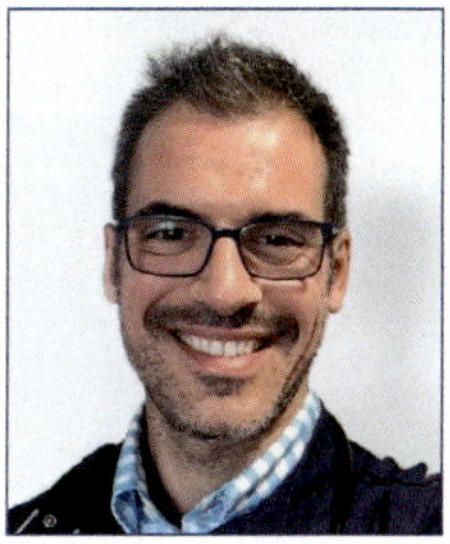

Fernando Martínez Taboada

Degree in veterinary medicine from Complutense University of Madrid in the year 2002. He completed an internship at the University of Bristol (United Kingdom) and then went on to do a residency in anaesthesia, analgesia and perioperative care at the same university. He became a certified specialist in veterinary anaesthesia by the Royal College Veterinary Surgeons (RCVS) in 2007 and has been a Diplomate if the European College of Veterinary Anaesthesia and Analgesia (ECVAA) since 2011.

He has worked as an anaesthesiologist and head of the anaesthesia and analgesia department at several academic and private referral centres in the United Kingdom and Australia. He currently combines his position as professor at the School of Veterinary Science of the University of Sydney (Australia) with his role as head of service at the Veterinary Teaching Hospital of the same institution.

He has been a speaker at congresses and training courses on the five continents and is a member of the Board of Directors of the Spanish Society of Veterinary Anaesthesia and Analgesia (SEAAV).

FOREWORD

Writing the foreword to this book is both a great honour and a great responsibility. This is because, despite the fact that the possible heart–kidney relationship had been glimpsed almost two centuries ago, it was little more than a decade ago in human medicine and three years ago in veterinary medicine when interest in the cardiorenal syndrome was renewed. This work is therefore likely to become an essential reading for veterinary surgeons.

The interpretation of concepts, definitions and nomenclature differ for veterinary medicine or human medicine. The pathophysiology of the cardiorenal syndrome is still at the stage of hypotheses in both fields. As the main target audience of this work are general veterinary surgeons, I think it is highly beneficial to make current knowledge more accessible so that they feel confident in applying it anywhere with the means they have at their disposal at the time.

For a better understanding of the syndrome, I will briefly review the knowledge acquired from the first suspicion of the heart–kidney relationship almost two centuries ago until the full identification and study of the cardiorenal syndrome in veterinary medicine.

Although the definitions and pathophysiology of the cardiorenal syndrome differ between veterinary and medical specialists in cardiology and nephrology, these all agree on the most important concepts: namely, that it is a syndrome, that it is an insufficiency syndrome, and that it can occur acutely or chronically.

Starting from the beginning, we should recall that the term “syndrome” is defined as a set of signs and symptoms that occur in different diseases. For example, icteric syndrome, anaemic syndrome, cyanotic syndrome, oedematous syndrome and, of course, cardiac insufficiency and renal insufficiency syndrome. “Insufficiency syndrome” is one in which the capacity of each organ to maintain homeostasis deteriorates. When the loss is sudden in a previously normally functioning organ, it would be a syndrome of acute organ failure, and when it occurs slowly and progressively, it would be a syndrome of chronic organ failure.

Focusing on the exciting history of the cardiorenal syndrome, we know that the first observation of the potential heart–kidney functional and pathological interrelationship was by Richard Bright, a physician at Guy’s Hospital in London from 1821 to 1843. One of my privileges to work and complete my nephrological training as Senior Registrar at the Chair of Nephrology, directed by the nephrology history enthusiast Professor J. S. Cameron, was, among others, direct access to the documentation kept at the hospital’s museum.

Dr Bright's first and most important findings were to identify the causes and consequences of kidney disease, his key finding being the discovery of the association between anasarca (*dropsy*) and proteinuria and nephrotic syndrome. Another finding (1836), probably the most interesting for us, was the relationship between cardiac hypertrophy and the course of kidney disease. However, he could not relate it to hypertension, as no technology was available at that time to quantify blood pressure. It was not until 1873 when Dr Frederick Akbar Mahomed, while still a student also at Guy's Hospital, began to work on the modification of the sphygmograph designed by Karl von Vierordt and modified by Étienne-Jules Marey until achieving a new quantitative sphygmograph model capable of measuring blood pressure in "troy ounces" (Mahomed, 1873), subsequently published by my mentor professor Cameron (Cameron and Hicks, 1996*)*. In addition, Dr Mahomed, in postmortem studies, was the first to correlate high blood pressure levels with cardiac hypertrophy, thickening and fibrosis of the arterial wall, aneurysms and damage to microcirculation (arteriocapillary fibrosis). He described most of the damaging effects of essential hypertension, giving it the name of "Bright's disease" without albuminuria, and later, hypertensive diathesis.

From this time until 2004, when cardiorenal syndrome was identified in human medicine, there are no references of interest. "Extreme cardiac and renal dysregulation" is then defined, leading to a syndromic entity in which treatment to alleviate clinical signs of congestive heart failure is limited by marked renal dysfunction. In 2008, it was redefined as "heart and kidney disorders, in which acute or chronic dysfunction in one organ induces acute or chronic dysfunction of the other".

In veterinary medicine, it is known that kidney and heart disease are a common cause of morbidity and mortality in dogs and cats, although heart–kidney interactions have received very little attention. Curiously, and interestingly, veterinary professionals, in my modest opinion, more aptly than physicians, propose the term "cardiovascular–renal axis disorders", consonant with the findings of Bright and Mahomed described, instead of the term "cardiorenal axis syndrome" used in human medicine. In 2015 veterinary professionals defined it as "a disease, structural or functional damage of the kidney, cardiovascular system, or both, induced by drugs or toxins, leading to an disruption of the normal interactions between these systems and causing the cardiovascular–renal axis disorder, identifying five subtypes, similar to those proposed in human medicine, depending on whether the primary cause is cardiac or renal and on the time of onset of damage".

As the main objective of this work is prevention, and if this is not possible, early diagnosis and treatment to prevent progression to stages with poorer prognosis, I will share with the reader the knowledge that have been most useful to me in daily clinical practice. For better understanding, it is important to remember the main functions of these two organs.

The primary function of the kidney is to maintain the balance of the internal environment. To achieve this, healthy kidneys must adjust the fluid and electrolyte balance, maintain the acid–base balance, regulate calcium–phosphorus mineral metabolism, modulate erythropoietin synthesis, perform tubular catabolism of some molecules, eliminate undesirable waste products from metabolism, and carry out glomerular filtration. The primary function of the heart is to infuse all organs with a constant, adequate blood flow to each organ to enable it to perform its functions. If cardiac function deteriorates to the point of being unable to maintain the required blood flow, the first clinical signs of dysfunction appear, which, if not identified and treated early, may progress from the preinjury stage to the injury stage within not more than a week. In the case of human medicine, it would also be affected by the age of the patient. In the elderly it would probably only require hours or days without treatment to occur. Thus, early interpretation of signs could indicate which of the organs is failing, the heart, the kidney, or both, and to act accordingly. Adding the above data to the medical history, physical examination and, if possible, an electrocardiogram and sometimes a chest X-ray, enables us to identify the aetiology and start adequate treatment to prevent progression to severe cardiorenal syndrome.

Finally, I would like to end the foreword to such a learned and comprehensive work – elaborated by members of the prestigious Animal Medicine Department of the Faculty of Veterinary Medicine of the University of Extremadura – to point out that research needs to be promoted. When I think about the importance and need for research, I mean basic research. Although it is important to deepen our knowledge of the pathophysiology of cardiovascular–renal disorders, the importance and need for research in clinical practice is no less important. More information is needed about essential aspects such as: the most common diseases in the different subtypes of the cardiorenal syndrome; the influence of age on their occurrence; the cardiac and renal functional grade that should alert us to prevent their onset; the cardiac and renal function threshold for the syndrome to appear and worsen; at what glomerular filtration rate it does so; what marker is better than serum creatinine due to variability between laboratories, even at the same centre; and if the phases and disease progression markers coincide with those in humans. In short, an exciting horizon of possibilities in veterinary medicine, for which I hope to have been able to awaken curiosity.

Juan Florencio Macías Núñez
Director of the extraordinary FIIPERVA Chair of the University of Salamanca: Iberoamerican Foundation for Prevention of Renal and Cardiovascular Disease

Salamanca, 15 May 2019

PREFACE

The main purpose of the book *Cardiovascular–renal axis disorders in dogs and cats* is to inform about the clinical repercussions that heart disorders can have on the kidney and vice versa in canine and feline medicine. This is intended to allow veterinary professionals to take into account such complications, as has been done in human medicine for several years, in order to achieve better results in the management of diseases related to both organs. The aim is for the book to be useful for small animal veterinary surgeons and for last-year veterinary students, by providing guidelines for the recognition of this type of disorder, as well as for the management of related complications.

The book begins with a chapter in which the different types of cardiorenal syndrome in human medicine are summarised, together with an update on the syndrome. Indeed, to better understand the bidirectional interaction pathways between the two organs in animals, it is very useful to know the advances in human medicine, pioneers in the study of these disorders.

A chapter with general considerations about the canine and feline species is then included, which reviews the current knowledge on this topic and the nomenclature adopted and prepares the reader to better understand the following chapters. These have been divided into several sections: the study of renal disorders that may occur as a result of cardiovascular diseases, cardiovascular disorders that may occur as a result of renal diseases, and situations in which both organ systems may be affected at the same time. Each chapter includes a definition of the disease in question, its pathophysiological study, the main diagnostic methods, and the recommended treatment.

Last, but not least, the book closes with a chapter focused on the anaesthetic management of patients with cardiovascular–renal axis disorders so veterinary surgeons can better prevent the anaesthetic complications due to these disorders.

This work aims to provide an up-to-date and practical view on a subject that will be increasingly important in veterinary medicine.

Javier Duque and Rafael Barrera
Editors

TABLE OF CONTENTS

01

CARDIORENAL SYNDROME IN HUMAN MEDICINE

M.ª Victoria Mogollón Jiménez • Gonzalo Marcos Gómez • David Chipayo Gonzales

Introduction

Since ancient times, several clinical conditions have been known in human medicine in which renal and cardiac damage or dysfunction occur simultaneously. However, it was not until 2004 when the National Heart Lung and Blood Institute coined the term cardiorenal syndrome (CRS) and defined it as "extreme cardiac and renal dysregulation", which leads to a syndrome in which treatment to relieve congestive clinical signs of heart failure (HF) is limited by marked renal dysfunction (NHLBI, 2014). A Consensus Conference was held in 2008 under the auspices of the Acute Dialysis Quality Initiative (ADQI), where the term CRS was defined as a series of "disorders of the heart and kidneys whereby acute or chronic dysfunction in one organ may induce acute or chronic dysfunction in the other organ". A 5-type classification was also proposed depending on the organ initially damaged and the acute or chronic nature of the damage (Ronco et al., 2008) (Table 1).

Recently, Hatamizadeh et al. proposed the bidirectional relationship of damage through haemodynamic, neurohumoral, and immunological pathways, an interaction supported by other recent studies (Bock and Gottlieb, 2010; Hatamizadeh et al., 2013).

Types of cardiorenal syndrome

Cardiorenal syndrome type 1 (CRS1)

Definition and epidemiology of CRS1

CRS1 refers to the condition in which acute cardiac dysfunction leads to acute kidney injury or dysfunction. Acute cardiac conditions that can lead to acute kidney injury include: acute heart failure, acute coronary syndrome, cardiogenic shock and disorders associated with heart surgery. CRS1 occurs in 25 % of patients hospitalised for acute decompensated heart failure (Dar and Cowie, 2008). Acute kidney injury (AKI) is an independent risk factor for mortality in patients with acute heart failure (AHF), including those with acute myocardial infarction (AMI) or reduced ejection fraction.

Table 1. Cardiorenal syndrome (CRS) classification.

Type	Denomination	Description
1	Acute cardiorenal	AHF leading to AKI
2	Chronic cardiorenal	CHF leading to CKD
3	Acute renocardiac	AKI leading to AHF
4	Chronic renocardiac	CKD leading to CHF
5	Systemic disease leading to heart and kidney failure	Systemic disease (sepsis, vasculitis) leading to AHF and AKI.

AHF, acute heart failure; AKI, acute kidney injury; CHF, chronic heart failure; CKD, chronic kidney disease.

Pathophysiology of CRS1

CRS1 is characterised by acute worsening of cardiac function (AMI, AHF) leading to AKI.

Haemodynamic changes play an important role in the pathogenesis of CRS1 in the presence of AHF, leading to decreased renal arterial flow and a consequent fall in glomerular filtration rate (GFR). These haemodynamic changes include not only impaired arterial flow as the cause of impaired glomerular filtration, but also congestive state (Prowle et al., 2010) and, for a long time now, increased intra-abdominal pressure (Winton, 1931) through an increase in venous pressure, which also causes an imbalance in glomerular flow and the subsequent impairment of glomerular filtration.

Among the nonhaemodynamic alterations, these patients also show activation of the renin–angiotensin–aldosterone system (RAAS) and the sympathetic nervous system (SNS). This causes vasoconstriction of the efferent and afferent arterioles, respectively, with a fall in renal blood flow, which amplifies the effect of the haemodynamic changes.

Similarly, chronic inflammation and imbalance in the production of reactive oxygen species (ROS) and nitric oxide (NO) (Heymes et al., 2003; Hornig et al., 2001; Kinugawa et al., 2000; Tojo et al., 2002; Vaziri et al., 2003) are involved in the pathogenesis of CRS1.

The iatrogenic effect in the pathophysiology of CRS1 should not be forgotten, with special mention of metformin and potentially cardiotoxic cancer drugs, which may also cause tubulointerstitial damage.

Diagnosis of CRS1

Early diagnosis of renal dysfunction is essential for adequate management of patients with CRS1. Traditionally, serum creatinine values have been one of the parameters used to define AKI. However, this classic marker rises when kidney injury is already established. Therefore, parameters that alert early to the existence of renal dysfunction are needed. Several molecules detectable in blood or urine with a greater predictive value for long-term death or rehospitalisation than creatinine or natriuretic peptides have been studied in recent years (Lassus et al., 2010) (see page 4).

It should be mentioned that all of these new markers are currently under investigation and while some of them such as cystatin C and neutrophil gelatinase-associated lipocalin (NGAL) seem to be promising, their measurement is not yet possible in all health services. With regard to clinical parameters, one of the most important ones in the evaluation of patients in whom AKI is suspected is urine output. Both this parameter and creatinine are studied in all risk assessment scales for AKI according to international recommendations, such as the Acute Kidney Injury Network (AKIN) classification (Table 2).

Echocardiography plays a major role in the diagnosis and scheduling of CRS1 management, as it can show the primary structural damage causing the syndrome (Di Lullo et al., 2012). Renal ultrasonography usually shows normal or slightly enlarged kidneys with preserved corticomedullary relationship, and Doppler ultrasound shows increased resistance with normal flow.

Classification of renal biomarkers

- Enzymes released by tubular cells: alkaline phosphatase, γ-glutamyl transpeptidase, alanine aminopeptidase, Ala-(Leu-Gly) aminopeptidase, fructose-1-6-biphosphatase, glutathione S-transferase isoenzymes α and π, N-acetyl-β-D-glucosaminidase.
- Low molecular weight molecules expressed in AKI: α-1-microglobulin, β-2-microglobulin, retinol binding protein, cystatin C, adenosine deaminase binding protein.
- Proteins specifically produced in the kidney under conditions of AKI: cysteine-rich protein 61, NGAL (neutrophil gelatinase-associated lipocalin), KIM-1 (kidney injury molecule-1), cytokines and chemokines such as Gro-α (growth-regulated oncogene α) and IL-18 (interleukin-18).
- Glomerular filtration rate markers: proatrial natriuretic peptide (pro-ANP), cystatin C.

Table 2. AKIN (Acute Kidney Injury Network) classification. This is the internationally accepted classification for the definition of acute kidney injury (AKI), as well as its staging according to severity.

AKI stages	Creatinine criterion	Urine output criterion
AKI 1	Creatinine increase ≥0.3 mg/dl or 1.5 times baseline	<0.5 ml/kg/h for 6 hours
AKI 2	Creatinine × 2 times baseline	<0.5 ml/kg/h for 12 hours
AKI 3	Creatinine × 3 times baseline or ≥ 4 mg/dl	<0.3 ml/kg/h for 24 hours or anuria for 12 hours

Treatment of CRS1

For the treatment of patients with AHF, particularly those with signs of tissue hypoperfusion, it is very important to identify those individuals at risk of developing CRS1. Implementation of appropriate preventive measures is a key strategy to reduce risks and improve patient prognosis.

Several clinical situations have been identified as predisposing risk factors for CRS1. Diabetes (Fig. 1), prior episodes of admission for decompensated heart failure or acute myocardial infarction, severe heart dysfunction, or impaired basal renal function are considered as nonmodifiable risk factors. Use of high doses of diuretics and vasodilator treatment, as well as high doses of radiographic contrast during invasive procedures, have been identified as modifiable risk factors.

Improving cardiac function and avoiding acute decompensation are the key elements of CRS1 prevention. Traditionally recommended measures include modifying cardiovascular risk factors, avoiding nephrotoxic agents

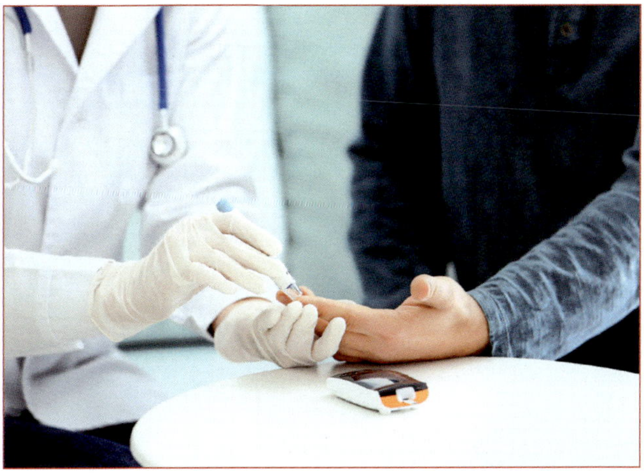

Figure 1. Assessment of blood glucose in a diabetic patient. Diabetes is a nonmodifiable risk factor that predisposes to cardiorenal syndrome type 1 (Africa Studio, Shutterstock.com).

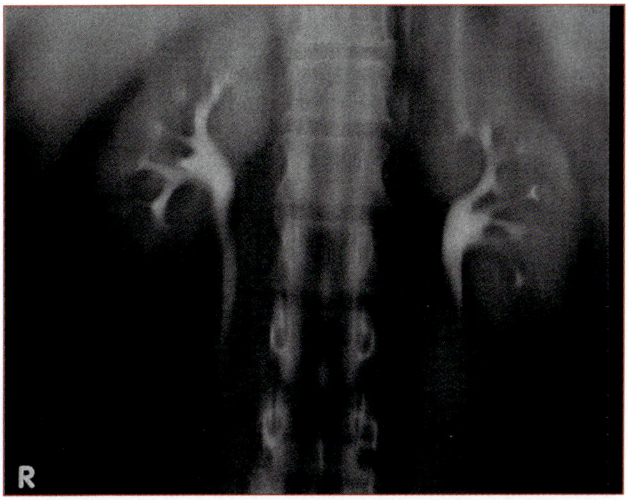

Figure 2. Iodinated contrast agents may act as nephrotoxic agents and contribute to the development of cardiorenal syndrome type 1 (Stefano Garau, Shutterstock.com).

and drugs that may favour salt retention, and appropriate pharmacological treatment of heart failure.

The nephrotoxic agents most commonly associated with the development of CRS1 are NSAIDs, thiazolindiones and iodinated radiological contrast agents (Fig. 2). NSAIDs and thiazolindiones act on renal haemodynamics and may lead to sodium retention and increased plasma volume. Iodinated contrast agents induce an intense and prolonged vasoconstriction in the corticomedullary junction of the kidney and impair the capacity of renal self-regulation; these effects, together with a direct tubular action, lead to acute tubular necrosis and the development of contrast-induced nephropathy.

If, despite our efforts, AKI classified as CRS1 develops, the main therapeutic objective will focus on the balance between the urine output required to control the patient's heart failure and the potential worsening of renal function due to volume loss and impaired perfusion.

Angiotensin-converting enzyme (ACE) inhibitors, angiotensin II receptor blockers (ARBs), and aldosterone antagonists are included in protocols for the management of heart failure because they have been shown to significantly improve survival in heart failure patients in randomised clinical trials (The Consensus Trial Study Group, 1987; Pfeffer et al., 1992; Pitt et al., 2003; The AIRE Study Investigators, 1993; Yusuf et al., 1991; Zannad et al., 2011). Some of them may contribute to the development of AKI due to impaired systemic and renal haemodynamics, so strict monitoring of both urine output and heart and kidney function will be required.

Diuretics are the first-line drugs in the treatment of patients with heart failure and CRS1. Congestion not only causes clinical signs but likely contributes to myocardial remodelling and progression of heart failure.

The optimal diuretic treatment regimen is unknown. No significant differences have been found in clinical signs or renal function depending on how the diuretic is administered, either as a bolus or as a continuous infusion, and at low or high doses (Felker et al., 2011). The high-dose approach has been associated with increased urine output and a more favourable prognosis in some secondary variables, but also with transient worsening of renal function. Loop diuretics predispose patients to electrolyte disturbances and hypovolaemia that can lead to neurohumoral activation and AKI. Hypovolaemia induced by the administration of diuretics can cause an increase in tubular sodium reabsorption and reduce response to these agents, particularly in patients with CKD.

Beta-blockers should be used with caution in patients with CRS1 and should in fact be avoided until the patient has been stabilised. This is because, in these situations, cardiac output is maintained by activation of the sympathetic nervous system and reflex tachycardia, so slowing this compensatory response may precipitate cardiogenic shock. In addition, introduction of RAAS-blocking agents should be performed by progressive dosing due to the associated risk of glomerular filtration impairment.

Inotropes (primarily dobutamine and levosimendan) may be useful in critically ill patients with volume overload resistant to diuretics and renal or liver dysfunction.

Renal replacement therapy (RRT) in these patients is an option when previous therapies have failed and patients present with congestion refractory to diuretic therapy and potentially life-threatening water and electrolyte or metabolic disorders (Bart et al., 2012).

Cardiorenal syndrome type 2 (CRS2)

Definition and epidemiology of CRS2

CRS2 is characterised by chronic cardiac dysfunction secondary to a fall in GFR. Chronic heart and kidney disease usually coexist. Renal failure is present in a high proportion of patients with CHF, ranging from 45 % to 63 % across studies (Hebert et al., 2010).

Pathophysiology of CRS2

CRS2 is characterised by chronic, progressive deterioration of renal function in patients with CHF. Two assumptions are made:

- CHF and CKD are simultaneously present but it is not possible to determine the causal relationship between these conditions.
- CHF causes CKD or its decompensation.

Neurohormonal activation, renal hypoperfusion, atherosclerosis, systemic inflammation, and oxidative stress represent the most important pathophysiological mechanisms of CRS2. Similarly, as in CRS1, chronic elevation of intra-abdominal pressure and systemic venous congestion play an important pathophysiological role. In experimental studies (D'Agati et al., 2011), a reduction in renal plasma flow together with persistent high intraglomerular pressure (for more than 6 months) caused podocyte damage, segmental glomerulosclerosis and, consequently, a progressive decline in GFR.

Diagnosis of CRS2

Damage is initially assessed by measuring creatinine levels, GFR, and renal protein excretion. Some biochemical markers (cystatin C, NGAL, KIM-1, and N-acetyl-β-D-glucosaminidase) have been evaluated in heart failure; their plasma levels may be used for the prognosis of cardiac failure, but are less useful to assess renal failure (Cruz et al., 2012).

An echocardiographic examination may again be relevant to diagnose the cause and thus guide treatment, together with a renal ultrasound, which will show a reduction in cortical thickness.

Treatment of CRS2

Treatment of heart failure is initially based on preventive aspects and control of cardiovascular risk factors.

One of the goals of heart failure treatment is to reduce volume accumulation without compromising cardiac output. Loop diuretics and thiazides, while they do not reduce mortality, improve clinical signs by reducing volume overload, and are recommended in patients with decompensated heart failure.

Beta-blockers (carvedilol, metoprolol, and bisoprolol) improve long-term ejection fraction and reduce mortality and rehospitalisation. Their efficacy has been proven in multiple randomised clinical trials (CIBIS-II, 1999; MERIT-HF, 1999; Packer et al., 1996).

As discussed in the previous section on CRS1, ACE inhibitors, ARBs, and mineralocorticoid receptor antagonists reduce morbidity and mortality in patients with CHF. However, ACE inhibitors and ARBs may reduce GFR, especially in the presence of diuretics and in patients with CKD or renal artery stenosis. The use of ACE inhibitors should be accompanied by careful monitoring of renal function and serum potassium levels due to the risk of hyperkalaemia, especially in patients with a concomitant renal dysfunction.

A new drug class consisting of therapeutic vehicles in supramolecular structures including an angiontensin II receptor antoganist (AIIRA) and a neprilysin inhibitor, an enzyme that degrades natriuretic peptides, has recently been shown to be effective and safe for treating patients with heart failure (McMurray et al., 2014; Velazquez et al., 2018).

In addition to drug treatment, implantable devices such as cardiac defibrillators and resynchronisation therapy are used in patients with heart failure with very specific indications, which are out of the scope of this chapter.

Cardiorenal syndrome type 3 (CRS3)

Definition and epidemiology of CRS3

CRS3, also defined as acute renocardiac syndrome, occurs when there is an abrupt worsening of kidney function, classified as either acute kidney injury (AKI) or acute renal failure, according to AKIN (Acute Kidney Injury Network) or KDIGO (Kidney Disease Improving Global Outcomes) diagnostic criteria, followed by acute heart failure (Kellum et al., 2012; Mehta et al., 2007).

CRS3 appears to be less common than CRS1, although its epidemiology is less well understood (Susantitaphong et al., 2013). AKI is a growing disorder in hospitals (Uchino et al., 2005). When the KDIGO criteria are applied, AKI is identified in approximately 20 % of hospitalised patients.

Pathophysiology of CRS3

The pathophysiology of CRS3 is not as well known as that of CRS1. The effect of AKI on the heart may be direct or indirect (Chuasuwan and Kellum, 2012).

Direct effects of AKI include both neuroendocrine and immune system activation. Sympathetic nervous system activation and noradrenaline release may have a direct harmful effect on the myocardial muscle (Singh et al., 2001), but also causes activation of the RAAS. Angiotensin II contributes to myocyte hypertrophy and modifies intracellular pathways involved in oxidative stress and inflammation (Kim and Iwao, 2000).

In addition, AKI stimulates immune system activation; in animal models it has been shown to increase the release of proinflammatory factors, accompanied by evidence of cardiac cell apoptosis (Kinsey et al., 2008). It may also have an indirect effect on the heart. Volume overload may lead to cardiac overload and pulmonary oedema; hyperkalaemia and other electrolyte disturbances may lead to cardiac arrhythmia and accumulation of uraemic toxins may decrease myocardial contractility and lead to pericardial inflammation and pericardial effusion (Meyer et al., 2007).

Diagnosis of CRS3

The diagnosis is again based on markers of kidney injury, which provide not only diagnostic but also prognostic information on CRS3, as well as on imaging techniques that give both renal and cardiac information.

NGAL appears to play an important role in the limitation of oxidative damage in acute and chronic renal failure, and represents a marker of early ischaemic damage. The kidney injury molecule (KIM-1) is a marker of ischaemic or toxic tubular injury. There are other markers such as liver-type fatty acid binding protein (L-FABP), IL-8, or netrin-1, but their clinical value has not been clearly demonstrated (Lassus et al., 2010).

As regards cardiac markers, the B-type natriuretic peptide (BNP) and N-terminal proBNP (NT-proBNP) as well as their ratio continue to be the best diagnostic and prognostic options. Troponins and heart-type fatty acid-binding protein (H-FABP) are other useful markers for diagnosis and prognosis in patients with renal failure (Lassus et al., 2010).

Treatment of CRS3

Prevention is the main strategy to reduce the consequences of CRS3. Thus, in patients at risk, it is advisable to avoid or reduce nephrotoxic drugs and ensure adequate hydration (Vanmassenhove et al., 2017).

In CRS3 it is important to look for the cause of AKI in case it has a specific treatment and to control complications. Adequate volume management is essential to prevent water overload, as well as treatment of electrolyte disturbances to prevent arrhythmia. In cases in which medical management is not sufficient, RRT may be considered (Bellomo et al., 2012) (Fig. 3).

Cardiorenal syndrome type 4 (CRS4)

Definition and epidemiology of CRS4

CRS4 is defined as the condition in which cardiovascular damage is associated with chronic renal failure that precipitates or is coadjuvant to cardiovascular impairment.

As in CRS2, there is a wide overlap in the timing and causes of worsening of both cardiovascular and renal injury due to the presence of common risk factors.

Heart disease is highly prevalent in patients with chronic kidney disease and the latter is a clearly accepted risk factor for the development of cardiovascular diseases, even more than for progression to end-stage chronic kidney disease (Coresh et al., 2004; Culleton et al., 1999; Go et al., 2004).

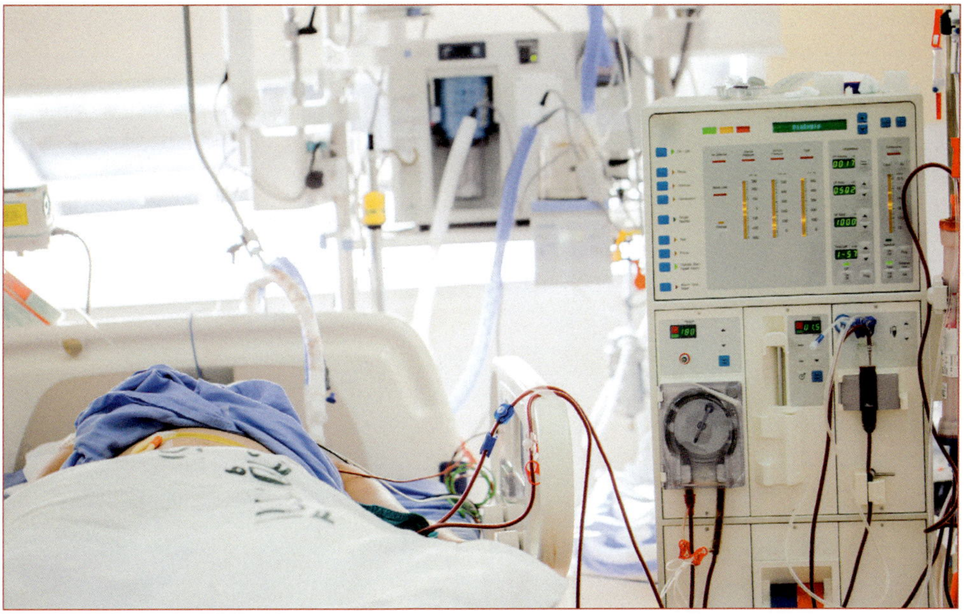

Figure 3. Advanced hospital dialysis equipment (Chaikom, Shutterstock.com).

Half of patients with advanced or end-stage renal disease (ESRD) die from cardiovascular causes (Di Lullo et al., 2015; Herzog et al., 1998; Tonelli et al., 2006).

Pathophysiology of CRS4

The pathophysiological process that would explain the association of CKD with the development of cardiovascular disease is complex (Dikow et al., 2005; González Maqueda, 2007).

Traditional risk factors are insufficient to explain the high prevalence of cardiovascular disease in the chronic kidney disease population.

When GFR falls below 60 ml/min, alterations occur in many physiological and regulatory functions. Thus, other nontraditional risk factors related to CKD have been shown to contribute to the development of cardiovascular disease, including anaemia secondary to an impaired erythropoietin synthesis, oxidative stress, impaired calcium-phosphorus metabolism, and accumulation of uraemic toxins (Muntner et al., 2005).

Hypertension is a potent cardiovascular risk factor for both the development of cardiovascular disease and CKD (Fig. 4). RAAS activation and sodium retention are major factors in the rise in blood pressure in the nephron (Guyton and Coleman, 1999).

Left ventricular hypertrophy, highly prevalent in haemodialysis patients, is a risk factor for the development of heart failure (Brenner et al., 2001).

Abnormalities in calcium-phosphorus metabolism are associated with progression of CKD and the development of cardiovascular complications. Hyperphosphataemia and secondary hyperparathyroidism, together with hypertension, promote calcification of cardiac vessels and valves. All of this contributes to atrial fibrillation and other types of arrhythmia.

Treatment of CRS4

Management of CKD should include compliance with dietary measures such as restriction of sodium, potassium, and protein intake. Control of traditional risk factors interfering with both conditions is also important, such as adequate blood glucose and blood pressure control. Blood pressure should be controlled using ACE inhibitors, ARBs, or beta-blockers due to their proven cardioprotective effects (Cice et al., 2003; Lewis et al., 2001).

As regards all other factors involved in the development of CRS4, metabolic acidosis should be treated by administration of sodium bicarbonate or sodium citrate. With regard to correction of anaemia, no clear advice is available, but administration of erythropoietin and iron in patients with heart failure is generally associated with improved heart and kidney function (Silverberg et al., 2000).

Cardiorenal syndrome type 5 (CRS5)

Definition and epidemiology of CRS5

CRS5 consists of acute or chronic renal and cardiac injury occurring simultaneously secondary to acute or chronic systemic disease. The most common cause is sepsis (Bagshaw et al., 2010), where concomitant cardiac and renal dysfunction are induced by proinflammatory cytokines, endotoxins, intrarenal and systemic vasodilation, increased vascular

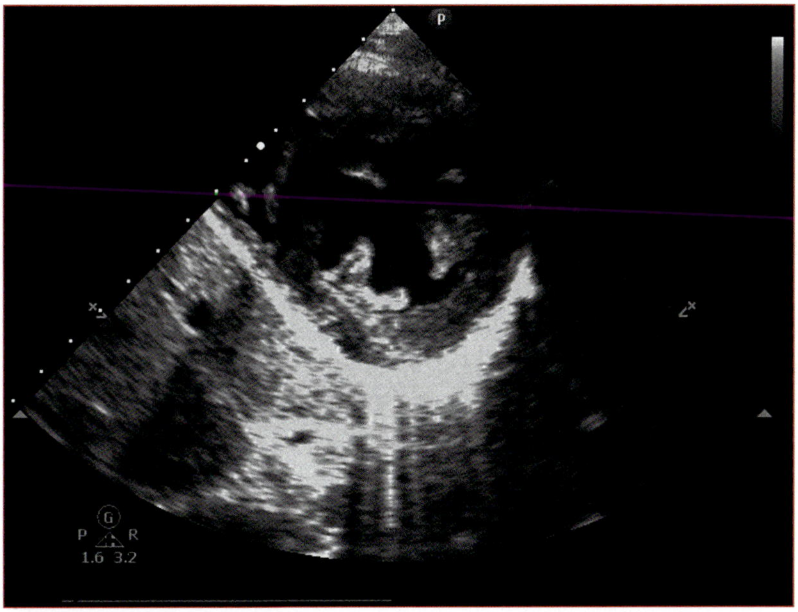

Figure 4. Standard two-dimensional transthoracic echocardiography in a patient with hypertension (Kalewa, Shutterstock.com).

permeability, hypoxia, and decreased perfusion. Other known causes of CRS5 include diabetes mellitus, systemic lupus erythematosus and other chronic inflammatory diseases (Abraham and Singer, 2007).

Pathophysiology of CRS5

The pathophysiology of CRS5 depends on the underlying disease and the speed of onset. Thus, several subtypes of CRS5 have been defined:

- Hyperacute (0–72 hours after diagnosis)
- Acute (3–7 days)
- Subacute (7–30 days)
- Chronic (over 30 days)

Diagnosis of CRS5

Diagnosis is based on an adequate history and physical examination taking into account previous comorbid conditions and risk factors that may contribute to the development of simultaneous cardiac and renal damage. Some markers of inflammation are useful for diagnosis (polysaccharide-linked protein, procalcitonin, C-reactive protein, IL-6, TGF-β) and imaging techniques such as echocardiography and renal ultrasound again provide information on underlying structural damage, predisposing to or precipitated by CRS5 (Di Lullo et al., 2012).

Treatment of CRS5

Treatment of CRS5 is based on the control of the cause and on supportive measures for renal and cardiac function. Intensive and early treatment of hypotension by volume provision and treatment with inotropic and vasopressor agents is important. As in other cases, when renal function is significantly reduced, RRT may be considered.

Conclusion

The existence of a physiological and pathophysiological interrelationship between the heart and kidney has been known since ancient times. However, it has only recently been classified, its pathophysiology and epidemiology studied, and therapeutic management organised.

Common risk factors in the development of renal and heart failure and the physiological interrelationship between both the cardiovascular and renal systems mean that the acute and chronic pathophysiological processes that affect them widely overlap.

The epidemiology is also affected by the high prevalence of cardiovascular risk factors and heart disease.

The diagnosis of CRS is based on an adequate clinical approach, which should include the medical history, physical examination and complex imaging techniques. Biochemical markers of damage that determine which of the organs is most affected and to what extent also play an increasingly important role.

Treatment is primarily based on adequate haemodynamic management for both maintenance of renal perfusion flow and adequate ventricular filling pressures, while also avoiding systemic venous congestion and increased intra-abdominal pressure. In many cases, treatment of the precipitating underlying cause, such as in acute CRS, is essential for adequate stabilisation of the patient.

Because of the overlap of renal and cardiac dysfunction, prevention of cardiovascular risk factors, which are the source of both acute and chronic kidney and heart disease, should not be forgotten.

02

OVERVIEW OF THE CARDIOVASCULAR–RENAL AXIS IN DOGS AND CATS

Javier Duque Carrasco • Rafael Barrera Chacón

Introduction

The heart and kidneys are functionally interconnected through the so-called "cardiorenal axis" (Fig. 1). This physiological connection occurs through several pathways, including renal perfusion pressure, heart filling pressure and neurohormonal activity. It is therefore logical to think that any alteration in one of these two systems may have clinical repercussions on the other, and vice versa. For example, a patient with heart failure will experience a decrease in cardiac output and systemic blood pressure, which will have a negative impact on kidney perfusion, leading to a deterioration in kidney function. On the other hand, if the kidneys initially fail, heart function may be impaired through activation of the renin–angiotensin–aldosterone system (RAAS) and sympathetic nervous system, development of hypertension (one of its target organs being the heart), or occurrence of arrhythmias due to electrolyte changes.

Dr Richard Bright first described the strong association between heart and kidney disease in human medicine in 1827. Since then, research has been ongoing. Interactions between the heart and kidney have now become an area of considerable interest, given their interdependence. This has led to the definition and conceptualisation of the "cardiorenal syndrome", which includes bidirectional interactions, where both acute and chronic alterations of either organ can affect either renal or ventricular function.

In 2008, Ronco et al. considered various scenarios for this syndrome, in which acute or chronic primary organ failure can be due to either the heart or the

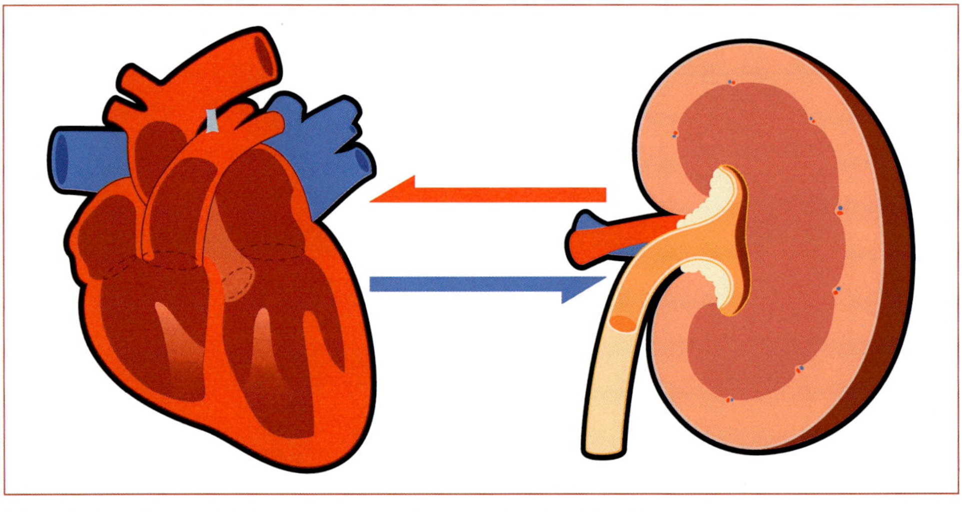

Figure 1. There is a physiological connection between the heart and the kidneys.

kidneys. The direct and indirect effects of functional alteration of each organ may initiate and perpetuate the damage to the other. To simplify these concepts in the clinical setting, a classification was established which divides the "cardiorenal syndrome" into five subtypes, considering the bidirectional (cardiac and renal) nature of the syndrome, the time frame of onset of damage (acute or chronic) and whether the primary cause is kidney disease, heart disease, or whether there is any multifactorial systemic disease causing heart and renal failure.

Although heart and kidney diseases in both dogs and cats are recognised as common causes of morbidity and mortality in veterinary medicine, the interaction between the two systems has not yet been studied in depth. In this regard, in 2015, a group of veterinary cardiologists and nephrologists from Europe and the United States met to establish a consensus on the definition, pathophysiology, diagnosis, and treatment of disorders that affect the interaction between the renal and cardiovascular systems. First, the term "cardiovascular–renal axis disorders" was proposed instead of the "cardiorenal axis syndrome" used in human medicine, and it has been defined as a disease, structural or functional damage to the kidneys, cardiovascular system, or both, induced by drugs or toxins, resulting in an alteration of the normal interactions between these systems.

Due to the need to better understand the bidirectional pathways of interaction between both systems to adapt treatment to each particular clinical condition, and based on the pathophysiological mechanism leading to cardiovascular–renal axis disorders, the expert group described five subtypes, conceptually similar to those proposed in human medicine, depending on whether the primary cause is cardiac or renal and the time frame of onset of damage.

Pathophysiology

The pathophysiological basis for this condition is still not well known, although several theories have been proposed that may explain the connection between heart disease and kidney disease (Fig. 2).

On the one hand, inadequate RAAS activation appears to play an important role in the development of both kidney and heart disease, as it results in increased sodium and water reabsorption, which is partly responsible for the development of heart failure. On the other hand, RAAS activation will lead to structural changes, such as myocardial remodelling, and promote fibrosis of both kidney and heart structure.

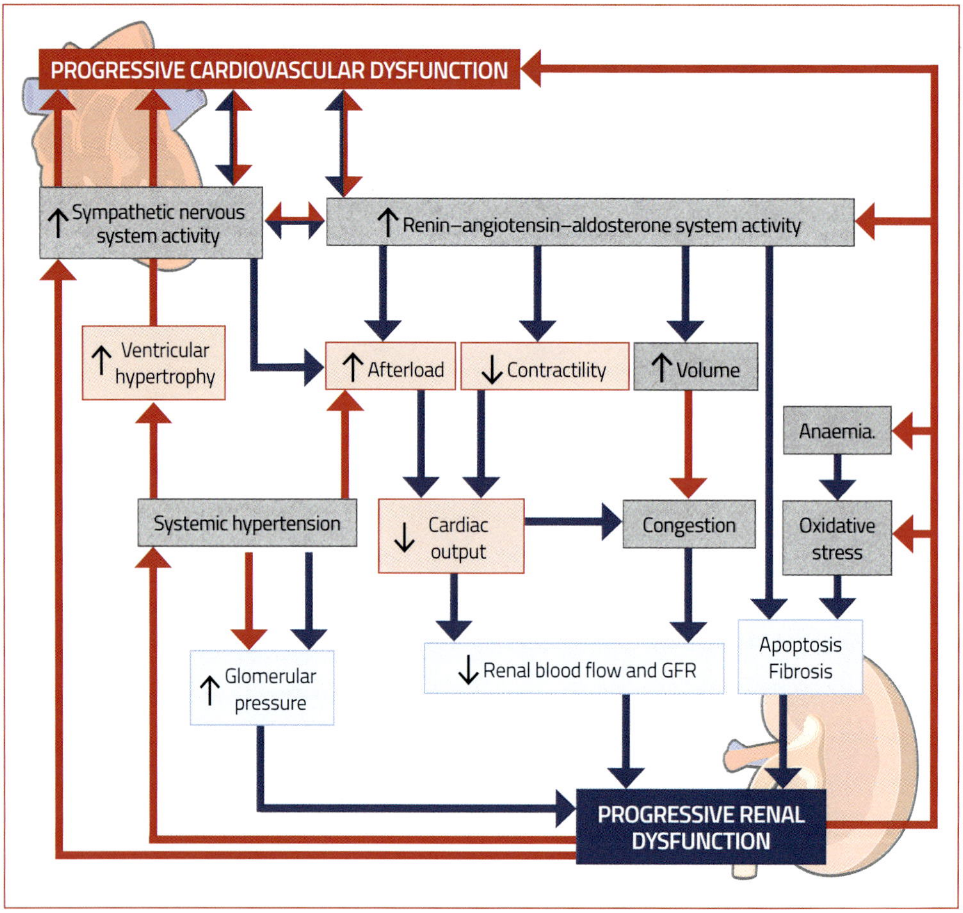

Figure 2. Mechanisms postulated to be responsible for the relationship between cardiac and renal dysfunction. Blue arrows: mechanisms by which heart disease can lead to kidney disease. Red arrows: mechanisms by which kidney disease can lead to heart disease (adapted from Pouchelon et al., 2015).

Other mechanisms involved in the development of cardiovascular–renal axis disorders include the following:

- Alteration of the balance between nitric oxide and oxygen free radicals. Nitric oxide leads to vasodilation and stimulates sodium excretion via the urine, while free radicals have opposite effects (sodium retention and renal vasoconstriction) and contribute to the development of hypertension. In cardiovascular–renal axis disorders, an imbalance occurs in favour of free radicals. Subsequent perpetuation of vasoconstriction causes significant tubular damage interfering with RAAS control mechanisms.

- Stimulation of factors involved in inflammation occurs in both heart and kidney failure, with an increase in several inflammatory mediators, such as tumour necrosis factor (TNF), interleukin-6 (IL-6), or C-reactive protein (CRP).
- Stimulation of the sympathetic nervous system in both heart and kidney disease leads to increased renin production, free radical generation and can induce inflammation.
- Anaemia appears to play an important role in this heart–kidney connection (some human medicine authors speak of the cardiorenal anaemia syndrome). Thus, anaemia may produce a state of cardiac hypoxia that causes the death of cardiomyocytes, leading to pathological remodelling of the heart, and in turn, to oxidative stress that contributes to this cell damage and stimulates the RAAS. Likewise, heart failure can cause anaemia as it contributes to impaired kidney function.

Classification

The bidirectional nature of cardiac and renal damage, the mutual interaction of these organs in haemodynamic regulation and the knowledge that other mechanisms are present in the development of the syndrome confer great complexity to the condition. To better understand this connection in human medicine, Ronco et al. (2008) classified the cardiorenal syndrome into five pathophysiological entities (Table 1): type 1 (acute cardiorenal syndrome), type 2 (chronic cardiorenal syndrome), type 3 (acute renocardiac syndrome), type 4 (chronic renocardiac syndrome), and type 5 (secondary cardiorenal syndrome). As discussed above, an equivalent classification (Table 1) established by a panel of experts of veterinary nephrologists and cardiologists is described below (Pouchelon et al., 2015.):

- Cardiovascular–renal disorders secondary to acute heart disease ($CvRD_{AH}$).
- Cardiovascular–renal disorders secondary to chronic heart disease ($CvRD_{CH}$).
- Cardiovascular–renal disorders secondary to acute kidney disease ($CvRD_{AK}$).
- Cardiovascular–renal disorders secondary to chronic kidney disease ($CvRD_{CK}$).
- Cardiovascular–renal disorders secondary to concomitant cardiac and renal diseases ($CvRD_{HK}$).

Table 1. Classification of cardiorenal syndrome in human and veterinary medicine.

Type of cardiorenal syndrome (human classification)	Consensus CvRD	Brief definition	Pathological processes
Type 1: Acute cardiorenal syndrome	**Unstable $CvRD_H$**	Acute worsening of cardiac function leading to acute kidney injury (AKI)	■ Acute heart failure ■ Cardiogenic shock
Type 2: Chronic cardiorenal syndrome	**Stable $CvRD_H$**	Chronic cardiovascular disease leading to progressive chronic kidney disease (CKD)	■ Chronic heart failure ■ "Congestive kidney disease"
Type 3: Acute renocardiac syndrome	**Unstable $CvRD_K$**	Acute primary worsening of renal function leading to cardiac dysfunction	■ AKI ■ Hyperkalaemia ■ Uraemia
Type 4: Chronic renocardiac syndrome	**Stable $CvRD_K$**	Primary CKD contributing to cardiac dysfunction	■ Chronic glomerular disease ■ Anaemia ■ Systemic hypertension
Type 5: Secondary cardiorenal syndrome	**$CvRD_O$**	Cardiac and renal dysfunction secondary to acute or chronic systemic disease	■ Diabetes mellitus ■ Sepsis

Unstable $CvRD_H$: cardiovascular–renal disorders secondary to acute cardiovascular disease.
Stable $CvRD_H$: cardiovascular–renal disorders secondary to chronic cardiovascular disease.
Unstable $CvRD_K$: cardiovascular–renal disorders secondary to acute renal disease.
Stable $CvRD_K$: cardiovascular–renal disorders secondary to chronic renal disease.
$CvRD_O$: cardiovascular and renal disorders secondary to concomitant heart and kidney diseases.
De Orvalho et al., 2017.

Cardiovascular–renal disorders secondary to acute heart disease ($CvRD_{AH}$)

These disorders are characterised by a rapid deterioration of cardiac function leading to acute kidney injury.

Pathophysiology

The pathophysiological mechanisms leading to acute kidney injury (AKI) in patients with acute heart failure are not fully understood, and the following have been suggested:

- Hypoperfusion caused by decreased cardiac output, which will result in an increase in laboratory parameters of kidney disease, but without structural damage in the kidneys, with prerenal azotaemia. This situation may evolve until, if left untreated, renal damage is established in the patient and perpetuated by low cardiac output. Cardiac dysfunction associated with haemodynamic

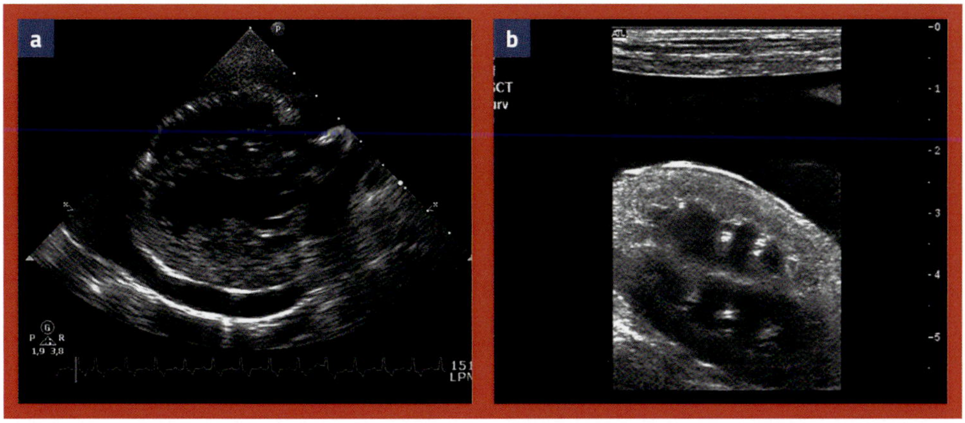

Figure 3. Echocardiography of a dog with pericardial effusion and secondary ascites (a). Congestion of the kidneys during heart failure has been proposed as a cause of cardiovascular and renal dysfunction secondary to heart disease (b).

worsening leads to activation of the body's compensatory mechanisms, in which the kidneys play a key role in regulating homeostasis of circulating volume and electrolytes. In this regard, the RAAS and the sympathetic nervous system play an important role in the genesis and progression of heart failure; activation of these systems is related to renal dysfunction.

- Renal venous congestion was proposed by members of the expert panel as a possible cause (Fig. 3). Increased central venous pressure may cause elevation of interstitial renal pressure due to retrograde transmission of right atrial pressure into the renal veins, which may result in a state of hypoxia in the renal parenchyma.
- Administration of certain drugs. Use of loop diuretics in patients with acute heart failure is essential (Fig. 4), but it predisposes to electrolyte disturbances and hypovolaemia, leading to neurohormonal activation and AKI.

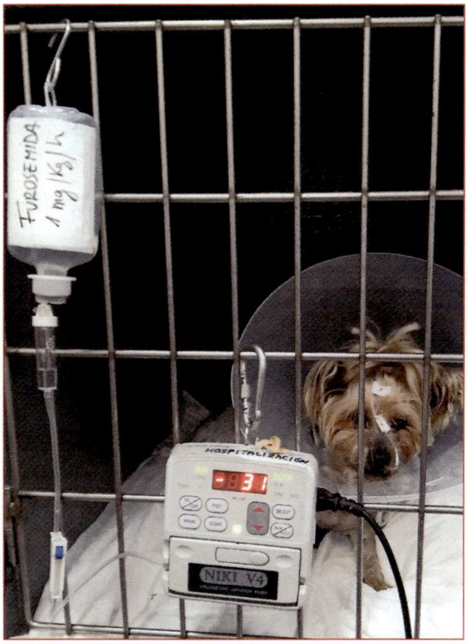

Figure 4. Hospitalised dog with pulmonary oedema due to heart failure secondary to mitral valve degeneration stage C (ACVIM). Administration of continuous infusion of furosemide. Loop diuretics, used routinely in heart failure, can lead to electrolyte disturbances and hypovolaemia, which will have a negative impact on renal function.

Causes of $CvRD_{AH}$

- Acute cardiac dysfunction leading to acute kidney injury.
- Acute cardiac dysfunction leading to acute renal dysfunction in patients with pre-existing chronic kidney disease.
- Decompensation of chronic heart failure causing acute kidney injury.
- Decompensation of chronic heart failure causing acute kidney injury in a patient with pre-existing kidney disease.
- Arterial thromboembolism leading to renal infarction.

Diagnostic tests

They are based on both laboratory data and diagnostic imaging methods:

- **Imaging diagnosis.** X-ray examination of the chest (Fig. 5) and echocardiography are two key pillars in the diagnosis of acute heart failure. The chest X-ray provides information on changes in the cardiac silhouette, vascular structures, and normal pulmonary pattern, and echocardiography is useful in the assessment of cardiac morphology and function. X-rays of the abdomen and ultrasound of the kidneys and urinary tract are recommended to detect morphological changes related to acute kidney injury.
- **Blood pressure measurement.** An important mechanism in the worsening renal function that can be observed in patients with acute heart failure is systemic hypotension, which occurs when systolic pressure falls below 90 mmHg. Measurement of this parameter is therefore essential for diagnosis and follow-up of cardiovascular and renal disease in these individuals (Fig. 6).
- **Laboratory tests.** The most commonly used cardiac biomarkers for diagnosis and follow-up of cardiovascular disease are troponin I and NT-proBNP (N-terminal fraction of brain or B-type natriuretic peptide). These markers are partially excreted by the kidneys; their values therefore depend on renal function and should be taken into account when evaluating patients with concomitant cardiac and renal dysfunction. Regarding AKI, it should be taken into account that this disorder of the cardiovascular–renal axis progresses rapidly, so that its early recognition represents a challenge for the veterinary professional. This is because the parameters commonly used to detect early stages of the disease according to the classification of the International Renal Interest Society (IRIS) (serum creatinine value and decreased urine output) are altered when the injury is already established in the kidney. Therefore, early warning biomarkers of renal dysfunction are needed (see below in the section corresponding to $CvRD_{AK}$).

Treatment

Treatment of this type of disorder of the cardiovascular–renal axis is aimed at developing strategies to improve cardiac output and renal perfusion pressure.

In order to increase cardiac output and thus ensure good renal perfusion, drugs such as pimobendan or intravenous infusion of dobutamine are used. Additionally, it should be noted that ACE inhibitors and high-dose

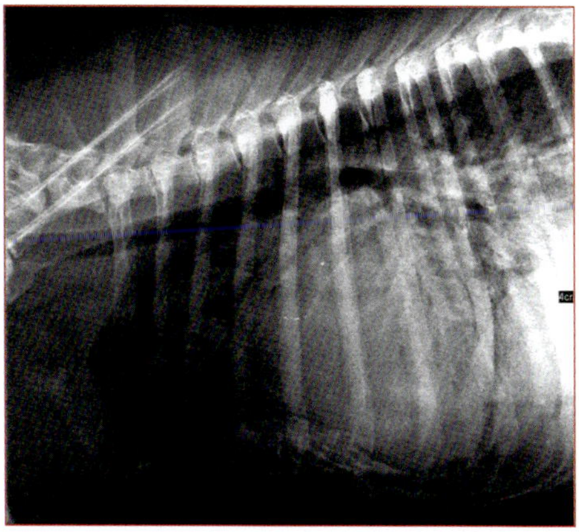

Figure 5. Lateral chest X-ray of a dog with pulmonary oedema due to heart failure.

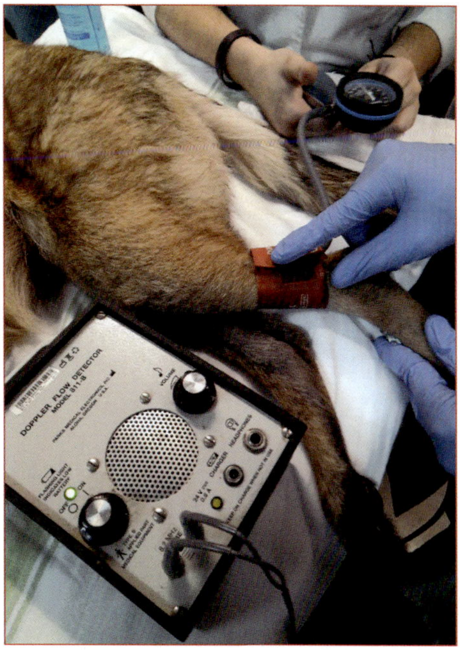

Figure 6. Measurement of systolic blood pressure in a dog using the Doppler method.

diuretics are indicated for the treatment of pulmonary congestion and oedema in these patients. However, treatment decisions including the use of these agents should consider minimising the risk of developing azotaemia by reducing daily parenteral diuretic administration, either by modifying the dose or frequency of administration, and using the lowest dose of ACE inhibitors in the therapeutic range.

If the animal is dehydrated after intensive administration of diuretics to treat acute heart failure, dehydration should be corrected by careful intake of intravenous or subcutaneous fluids, taking into account their sodium and potassium content.

Cardiovascular–renal disorders secondary to chronic heart disease ($CvRD_{CH}$)

These disorders present with the development of chronic congestive heart failure that can cause progressive and potentially permanent chronic kidney disease (CKD).

Pathophysiology

Although there is a very limited understanding of the pathophysiology of CKD in the setting of advanced chronic heart disease, it is clear that a chronically decreased cardiac output will cause, over a prolonged period of time, a state of hypotension and decreased renal perfusion, which will stimulate the following mechanisms:

- Compensatory neurohormonal response, which will result in activation of the RAAS and sympathetic nervous system, in addition to increased expression of molecules such as vasopressin, endothelin, and natriuretic peptides. Increased production of angiotensin II and aldosterone by the kidneys will promote water and sodium retention, which will cause hypertension. Angiotensin II will also produce high renal endothelin-1 levels, which will initiate and promote the progression of inflammation and fibrosis in the kidney. The high aldosterone levels together with angiotensin II will lead to the development of renal fibrosis and glomerular sclerosis.

- Chronic renal hypoxia will result in increased oxidative stress, which will cause worsening endothelial function and establishment of a chronic inflammatory state. Increased levels of tumour necrosis factor (TNF) and interleukins-1 and -6 (IL-1 and IL-6) related to the mentioned chronic inflammatory state will lead to progressive toxic damage and apoptosis of kidney cells, which will contribute to irreversible kidney damage and impairment of renal function.
- The study of anaemia (Fig. 7) in cardiovascular–renal axis disorders has recently gained great interest in human medicine. Thus, some studies refer to the cardiorenal anaemia syndrome, characterised by the presence of anaemia, chronic heart disease, and CKD. Anaemia appears to play a relevant role in the generation of a state of cardiac hypoxia.
- Finally, it is necessary to mention the treatment of heart failure as the cause for deterioration of renal function. Patients with chronic heart disease often receive long-term high doses of diuretics and vasodilators, which may lead to the development and progression of chronic kidney damage.

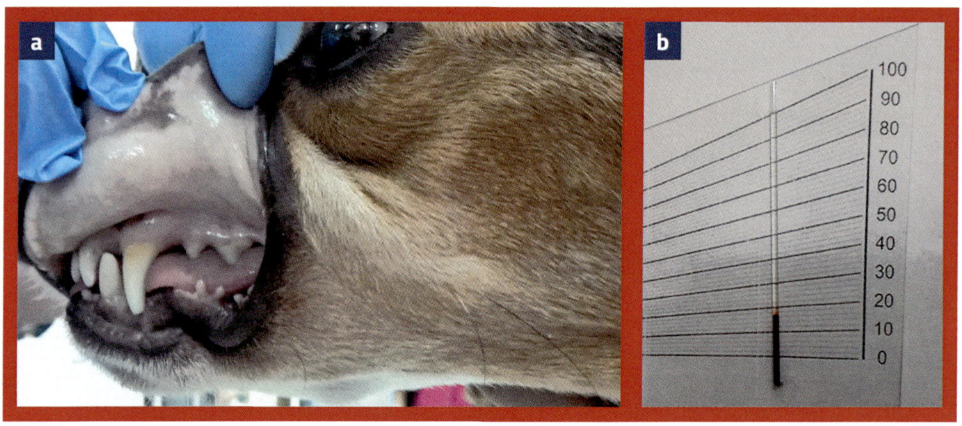

Figure 7. Pale mucous membranes (a) and decreased haematocrit (b) in a dog with anaemia; this appears to play an important role in the heart–kidney connection and some authors have even spoken of the cardiorenal anaemia syndrome.

Causes of $CvRD_{CH}$

- Systemic hypertension that may lead to glomerular disease.
- Congestion of the kidneys during heart failure.
- Renal hypoperfusion due to decreased cardiac output (Fig. 8).
- Filariosis or vena cava syndrome leading to the development of glomerular disease (Fig. 9).

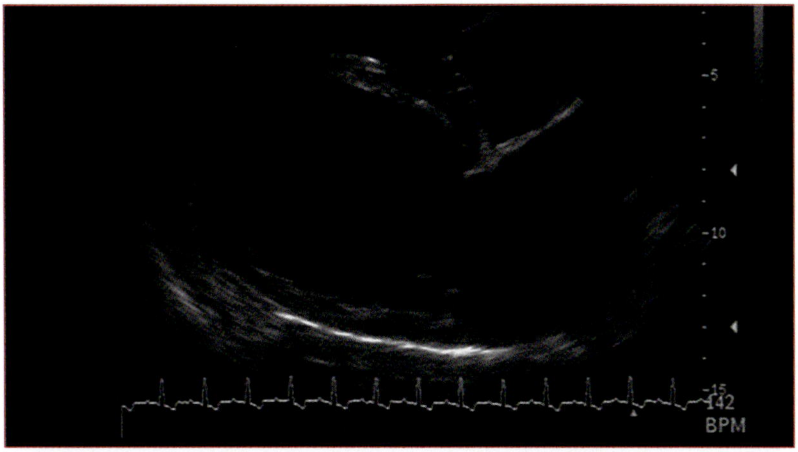

Figure 8. Echocardiography in a dog with dilated cardiomyopathy. Right parasternal long axis view. Cardiac output is decreased and renal hypoperfusion will occur.

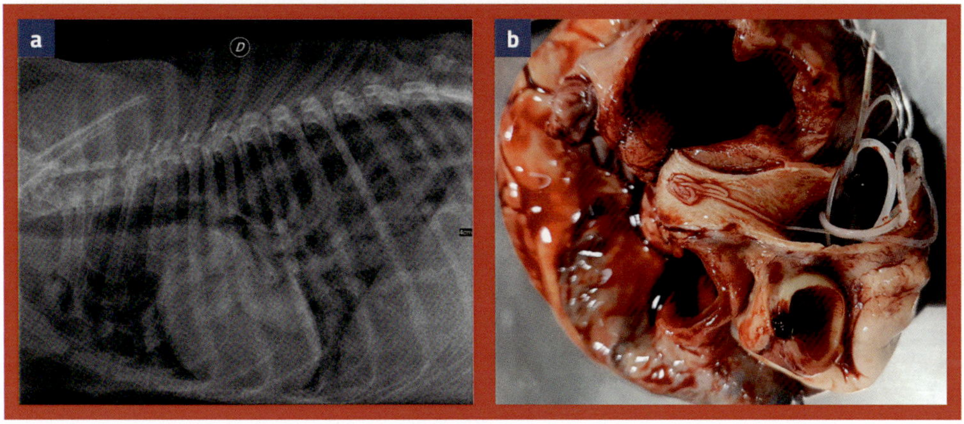

Figure 9. Lateral chest X-ray (dilation of pulmonary arteries) (a) and presence of adult *Dirofilaria immitis* worms in the pulmonary artery (postmortem study) of a dog with heartworm disease (b).

Diagnostic tests

Veterinary surgeons should use the different diagnostic tools available to them to first characterise heart disease and then evaluate its impact on renal function:

- **Imaging diagnosis.** Chest X-rays provide information on changes in the cardiac silhouette, as well as on pathological alterations in the vascular and pulmonary pattern. Echocardiography can be used to identify the patient's heart disease and establish the degree of cardiac dysfunction using different echocardiographic examination modalities, such as B-mode (Fig. 10), M-mode (Fig. 11) and Doppler (Fig. 12) (colour, spectral and tissue), as well as more advanced techniques such as deformation (strain) analysis, deformation rate (strain rate) and speckle tracking (2D speckle tracking). Abdominal ultrasound may be useful in detecting morphological changes in the kidneys and urinary tract related to CKD.
- **Laboratory tests.** The most commonly used cardiac biomarkers for evaluating and monitoring the progress of heart diseases are cardiac troponin I and B-type natriuretic peptide. It should be noted that these parameters show some weak points when used in a case of dysfunction affecting both the heart and kidneys, since their value may be increased both in heart disease and kidney disease. Some studies have shown significant "grey zones" that do not allow patient populations to be stratified based only on their determination (a range of values for these parameters may not always make it possible to distinguish normal from pathological). It is therefore sometimes difficult to know whether the increase in troponins and natriuretic peptides in dogs and cats reflect cardiac injury, normal variation, or a decrease in their excretion.

The fact that anaemia seems to have per se a relevant role in the pathogenesis of cardiovascular–renal axis disorders requires evaluation of at least red blood cells. In order to determine the impact that cardiac dysfunction may have on renal function, blood chemistry and urinalysis are recommended (see below under the sections for $CvRD_{AK}$ and $CvRD_{CK}$).

All these markers are sensitive for detecting renal damage, though their ability to differentiate between primary or secondary kidney disease and heart disease in the context of cardiovascular–renal axis disorders has not been tested. Therefore, the search for disease-specific markers is of great interest in both human and veterinary medicine.

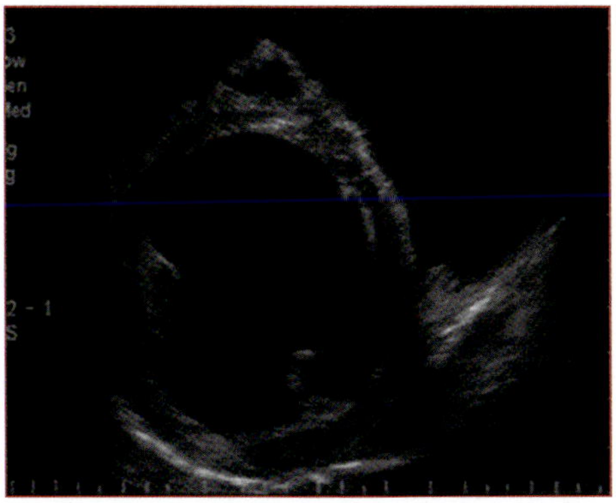

Figure 10. B-mode echocardiography in a dog, right parasternal short axis view of the left ventricle.

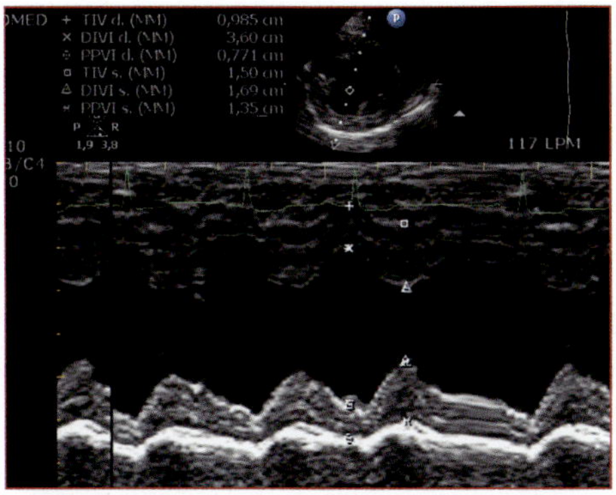

Figure 11. M-mode echocardiography of the left ventricle in a dog.

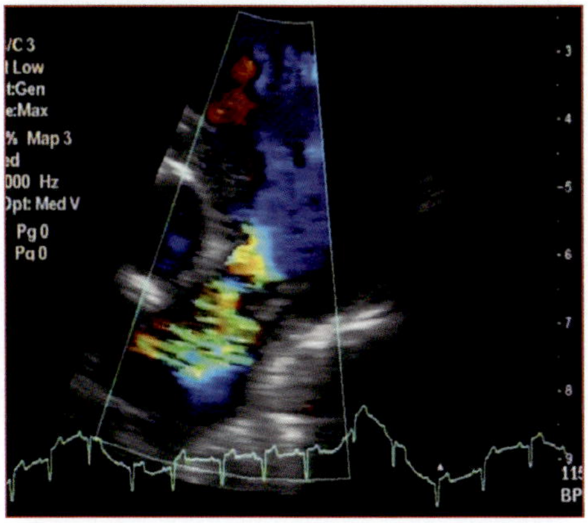

Figure 12. Colour Doppler echocardiography at the pulmonary valve level in a dog.

Treatment

Since the pathophysiological basis for this condition is very complex and often not well known, it should be considered that there is no defined treatment strategy.

Given that RAAS activation appears to be critical in the pathogenesis of this condition, it is logical to think that the use of drugs that block RAAS activation is of great importance. Thus, concomitant use of ACE inhibitors and angiotensin receptor blockers will protect both the heart and the kidney. In addition, the use of drugs that inhibit aldosterone facilitates management of these patients. Added to the protective effects of these drugs on both the heart and kidney are the benefits obtained from reducing blood pressure and the effect on reducing proteinuria, which could slow the progression of damage to the heart and kidneys.

The use of diuretics is essential to treat pulmonary congestion and oedema in these patients, but high doses are often used that contribute to renal injury due to excessive urine output. Therefore, care should be taken with this situation and strategies should be adopted to try to avoid or minimise this, such as the use of loop diuretics in continuous infusion or the combination of these with other agents with a different mechanism of action (e.g. thiazides).

Administration of pimobendan improves systolic function, which may increase glomerular filtration rate (GFR).

Correction of anaemia could be of interest in the management of these patients, as shown in human medicine.

Finally, use of an adequate diet may be decisive, as well as oral supplementation with omega-3 fatty acids acting as antioxidants and appetite stimulants, both in patients with kidney and heart disease.

Cardiovascular–renal disorders secondary to acute renal diseases ($CvRD_{AK}$)

These disorders are characterised by damage or dysfunction of the cardiovascular system secondary to acute diseases that primarily affect the kidneys. This can occur through multiple mechanisms, including volume overload, electrolyte disturbances, neurohormonal activation, and myocardial depressant factors. This may manifest as arrhythmias, pericarditis and acute heart failure. The IRIS classification is very useful for their evaluation.

There is not yet much evidence of this association in canine and feline medicine, and, as in human medicine, the existing ones are not as numerous and are not as well established as in $CvRD_{AH}$ and $CvRD_{CH}$.

Pathophysiology

An established pathophysiological consequence in dogs with AKI is electrolyte abnormalities, mainly represented by hyperkalaemia, which may be associated with cardiac arrhythmia, and with a lower incidence due to hypokalaemia, sometimes common in the recovery phase of the disease. On the other hand, patients who suffer an AKI due to different causes and who previously had heart disease treated with drugs promoting renal excretion, such as digoxin, show a dramatically reduced elimination of these drugs, and may therefore develop signs of toxicity, including arrhythmia, hypotension and myocardial function disorders.

Patients with severe AKI often present with anorexia and dehydration due to not wanting to drink and vomiting. All this affects body fluid volume and consequently the haemodynamic status of the animal, reflected by a decrease in cardiac output.

Finally, acute failure of renal function may lead to volume overload that contributes to vascular congestion, particularly if the animal has coexisting prior heart diseases, such as valve disease, dilated cardiomyopathy, hypertrophic cardiomyopathy, hypertensive heart disease, and severe anaemia.

In human medicine, this syndrome is also associated with high levels of inflammatory mediators, such as tumour necrosis factor and interleukins, which alter cardiac function by affecting contractility and stimulating apoptosis in cardiomyocytes, in addition to systemic damage and high mortality.

Causes of $CvRD_{AK}$

- Hypokalaemia or hyperkalaemia (Fig. 13), which may be responsible for cardiac arrhythmias.
- Decreased renal clearance of drugs, such as digoxin, which may result in toxicity.
- Dehydration, which may lead to volume depletion and decreased cardiac output and tissue perfusion.
- Uraemic pericarditis.
- Activation of the renin–angiotensin–aldosterone system, responsible for sodium and water retention, cardiac and vascular remodelling, and congestion.

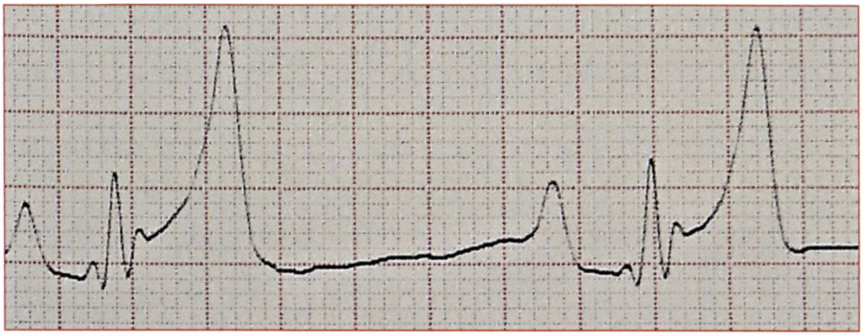

Figure 13. Electrocardiogram of a dog with hyperkalaemia; peaked T-waves are seen.

Diagnostic tests

Based on both laboratory data and diagnostic imaging techniques.

- **Diagnostic imaging.** Although the presence of AKI in dogs and cats is rarely associated with changes detectable by diagnostic imaging techniques, they are always required to both confirm and rule out certain diseases. A radiological study can provide information about the size and position of the kidneys, as well as the presence of uroliths (radiodense). Abdominal ultrasound allows visualisation of renal parenchyma abnormalities, dilations of the renal pelvis (Fig. 14) and ureters (Fig. 15), renal flow abnormalities, and the presence of uroliths, and helps in the diagnosis of pyelonephritis and ethylene glycol poisoning. More advanced techniques such as excretory urography, magnetic resonance imaging, or computed tomography are sometimes needed.
- **Blood pressure measurement.** Increased blood pressure is one of the best known mechanisms in the development of the cardiovascular–renal syndrome. Measurement is recommended in all cases of both acute and chronic

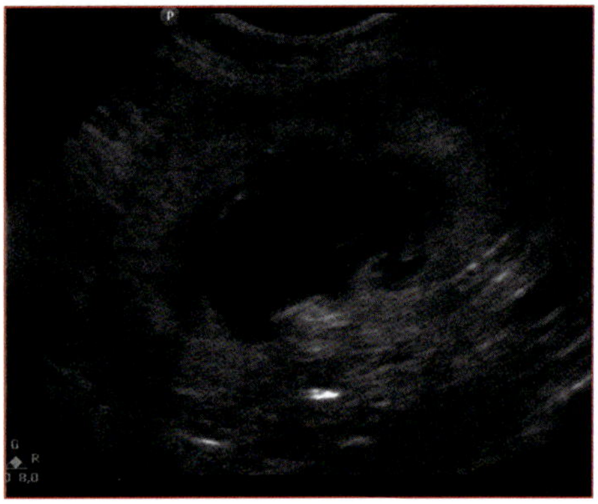

Figure 14. Enlargement of the renal pelvis in a cat due to the presence of uroliths in the ureter.

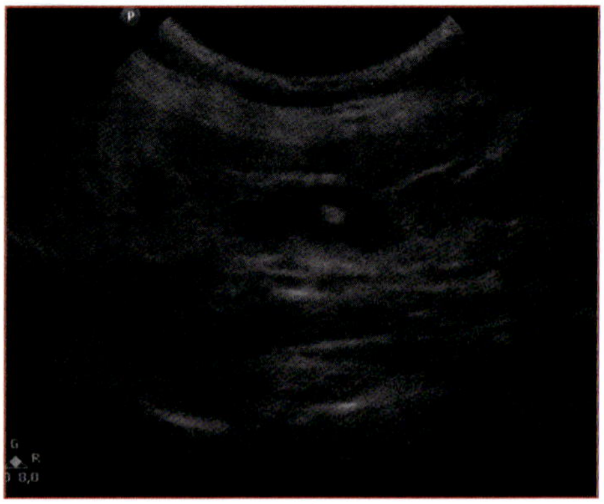

Figure 15. Ureteral enlargement and presence of a stone in the ureter of a cat.

kidney disease. Hypertension is a major risk factor for the development and progression of kidney disease (IRIS). In dogs, it is directly related to kidney damage, proteinuria, decreased GFR, worsening of uraemic crises, and increased mortality. In cats, the relationship between kidney disease and hypertension is less clear. Hypotension, for instance due to a volume reduction, reduces tissue perfusion and GFR, and activates maladaptive neurohormonal responses. When severe, it can lead to renal hypoperfusion with subsequent organ damage.

- **Laboratory tests.** Renal dysfunction (due to primary or secondary renal diseases) is characterised by having a wide range of laboratory biomarkers for its diagnosis (see next page). These are the ones used to diagnose cardiovascular–renal axis diseases to confirm the renal origin of the condition, accompanied by the previously described biomarkers of impaired cardiovascular function. To evaluate possible repercussions on the body's homeostasis, electrolyte levels (capacity to maintain electrolytes is evaluated) and bicarbonate levels (acid–base balance is evaluated) are usually measured in blood.

Finally, all diagnostic tests required to assess cardiac function should also be performed, as described above.

Treatment

Treatment of AKI typically requires hospitalisation of animals in order to restore fluid and electrolyte balance, while at the same time assessing the risk of cardiovascular dysfunction. Patients, once hydrated, often require treatment with diuretics to induce urine output, as well as antihypertensive agents. In this case, special care should be taken with the doses used, particularly in the case of loop diuretics such as furosemide.

Renal biomarkers

In general, biomarkers assess alterations in the glomerular filtration rate, urine concentration capacity, and tubular function, as well as the impact that altered renal function may have on the body's homeostasis.

Available biomarkers are divided into **classic** biomarkers, those most commonly used and studied, but also those that provide later information (especially important in CKD), and **novel** biomarkers, most of which are still being studied and are intended to detect kidney disease earlier.

The classic markers used for the assessment of glomerular filtration capacity are mainly the blood concentration of urea and creatinine, and also proteinuria. The microalbuminuria test, protein:creatinine ratio (or UPC ratio) and, more recently, immunoglobulin G concentration in urine are also used.

The concentrating ability of the kidney should preferably be evaluated by measuring urinary osmolality. However, because of the equipment required for its determination, urine density is usually used.

Biomarkers of tubular function are particularly important in the diagnosis of AKI, since these functional alterations are very specifically associated with this condition. Glycosuria has traditionally been used in the absence of hyperglycaemia, as well as the presence of cylindruria (Fig. 16). However, these findings are not common or sufficiently sensitive, and are therefore replaced by other laboratory measurements, most of which provide information about the status of the proximal segment of the renal tubule, and are measured in urine, such as: fractional excretion of electrolytes, N-acetyl-β-D-glucosaminidase or NAG, urinary cystatin C, retinol binding protein or RBP, γ-glutamyl transpeptidase or GGT, neutrophil gelatinase-associated lipocalin or NGAL, and clusterin.

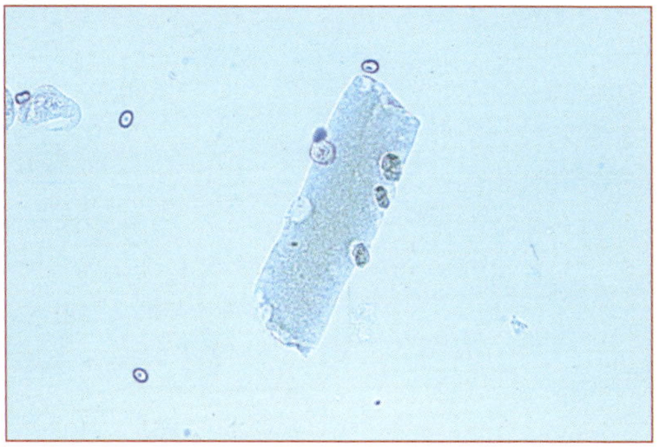

Figure 16. Cylinder in urine sediment of a dog. Cylindruria may be associated with acute kidney injury.

Cardiovascular–renal disorders secondary to chronic kidney disease ($CvRD_{CK}$)

These disorders are characterised by damage to or dysfunction of the cardiovascular system secondary to chronic diseases affecting the kidneys primarily, and leading to left ventricular hypertrophy, diastolic dysfunction, and increased risk of cardiovascular disease. As with AKI, there is also not much evidence of this association in canine and feline medicine.

Pathophysiology

This association between CKD and cardiovascular disorders is attributed to the presence of arrhythmias secondary to hyperkalaemia (less common than in AKI), toxicity due to a decreased excretion of drugs used in the treatment of cardiac diseases (e.g. digoxin and enalapril), decreased cardiac output in advanced renal disease (mainly due to dehydration), volume overload due to hypervolaemia in terminal oligoanuric phases of the disease and the effects of the anaemia often seen in these animals (though not a common pathophysiological process). In uraemic conditions, azotaemia may affect myocardial cells, altering their normal function. Finally, the association between hypertensive CKD and heart disease is important, because it may lead to the development of myocardial hypertrophy and cardiac dysfunction.

In its evaluation in dogs and cats, as with AKI, the classification established by the IRIS is very useful.

Causes of $CvRD_{CK}$

- Systemic hypertension of renal origin.
- Volume overload leading to systemic hypertension.
- Hypokalaemia or hyperkalemia, which may be responsible for cardiac arrhythmias.
- Decreased elimination of drugs, such as digoxin, which may cause toxicity.
- Dehydration, which may lead to volume depletion and decreased cardiac output and tissue perfusion.
- Uraemic pericarditis.
- Activation of the renin–angiotensin–aldosterone system, responsible for sodium and water retention, cardiac and vascular remodelling, and congestion.
- Anaemia may lead to volume overload and decreased oxygenation of cardiac tissue.

Diagnostic tests

As in the previous case, they would be based on:

- **Diagnostic imaging.** It is similar to that described for AKI. As with AKI, in dogs and cats there are often no renal changes detectable with diagnostic imaging techniques.
- **Blood pressure measurement.** It is very important in dogs and cats with CKD. Particularly because of its relationship with proteinuria (Fig. 17), a very common finding in glomerular diseases. Hypertension is a risk factor for proteinuria, which in turn is a factor related to progression of kidney disease.
- **Laboratory tests.** The laboratory biomarkers described for AKI are used. However, while it is true that early diagnosis is very important in both AKI and CKD, it becomes particularly important in the latter. In fact, the IRIS classification recommends in stages 1 and 2 to complete the diagnosis obtained by measurement of serum creatinine with measurement of serum symmetric dimethylarginine (SDMA), which allows for earlier diagnosis of glomerular disease. Other indicators of glomerular damage, such as plasma cystatin C, are still under study. Measurement of urinary density and the UP:C ratio is very important in this disease. Although tubular markers are associated with AKI, their determination in CKD is also relevant, because a glomerular process eventually becomes mixed (glomerular and tubular) and they can often be used as earlier biomarkers than serum urea and creatinine.

The diagnostic tests required to assess cardiac function should also be performed, as described above.

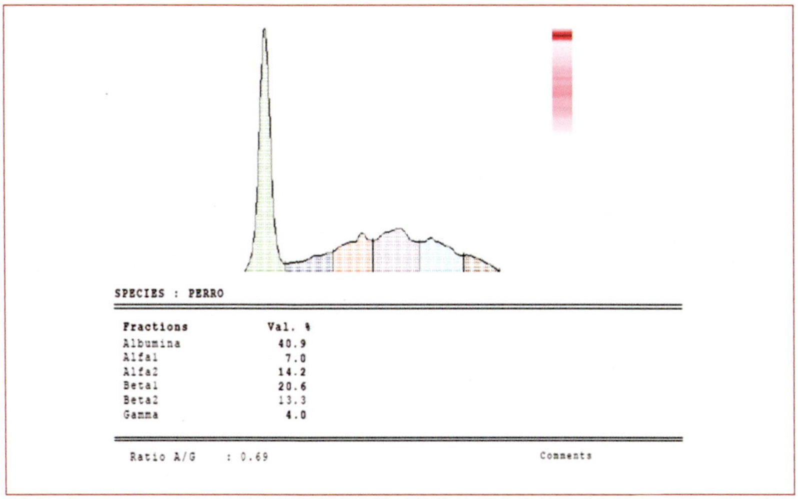

Figure 17. Urine electrophoresis of a dog with leishmaniasis for the study of proteinuria.

Treatment

It consists primarily of controlling CKD. It is very important to lower blood pressure in cases of hypertension and monitor the dose of antihypertensive drugs, as many of them are eliminated renally. It is also very important to perform laboratory tests for proteinuria and plasma phosphorus, which is indicative of advanced disease and survival. Dogs and cats with CKD have lower survival, so periodic monitoring should include examination of their cardiovascular function, and treatment completed based on the findings found.

Cardiovascular–renal disorders secondary to concomitant cardiac and renal diseases ($CvRD_{HK}$)

This syndrome is characterised by an acute or chronic systemic disease causing simultaneous cardiac and renal damage.

Pathophysiology

The pathophysiology of this type of cardiovascular–renal axis disorder, as well as the time frame over which it develops (acute or chronic), depend on the underlying cause. For example, in the case of sepsis, a fulminant process can occur with an acute impact on cardiac and renal function.

However, it should be noted that this interaction is currently poorly defined in dogs and cats, and further studies providing more scientific evidence are needed.

Causes of $CvRD_{HK}$

- Septic or neoplastic embolism causing renal (Fig. 18) and cardiac infarction.
- Gastric dilatation volvulus (Fig. 19) leading to arrhythmias and azotaemia.
- Parasitic diseases (*Trypanosoma cruzi, Leishmania infantum*) (Fig. 20).
- Glycogen storage diseases that cause deposition of this polysaccharide in the heart and kidneys.
- Pancreatitis (Fig. 21).
- Hyperadrenocorticism (Fig. 22).
- Amyloidosis: patients with this disease may experience amyloid deposition in the heart and kidneys.

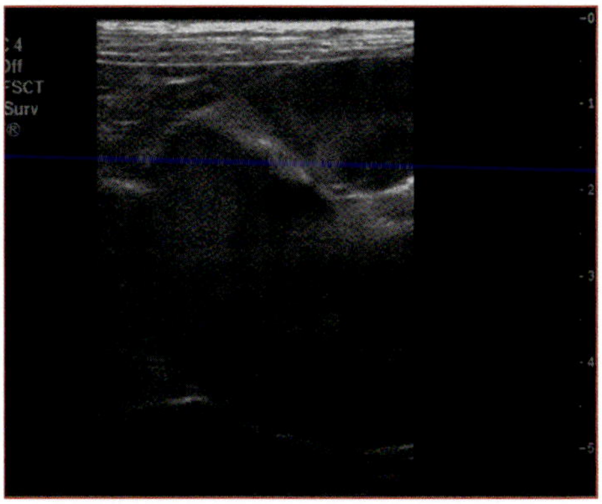

Figure 18. Renal ultrasonography of a dog where a hyperechoic cortical infarct of wedge-like appearance can be seen.

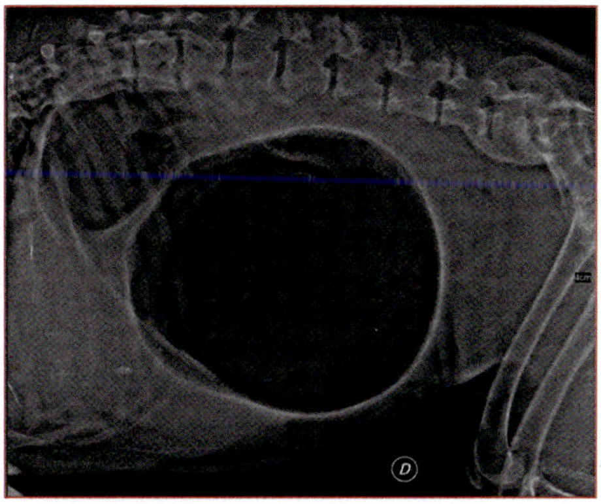

Figure 19. Lateral X-ray of abdomen of a dog with gastric dilatation volvulus.

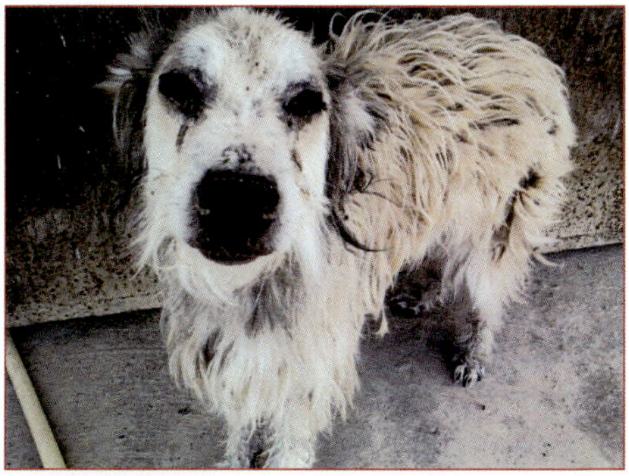

Figure 20. Dog with leishmaniasis. Myocarditis and chronic kidney disease may be seen concomitantly in these patients.

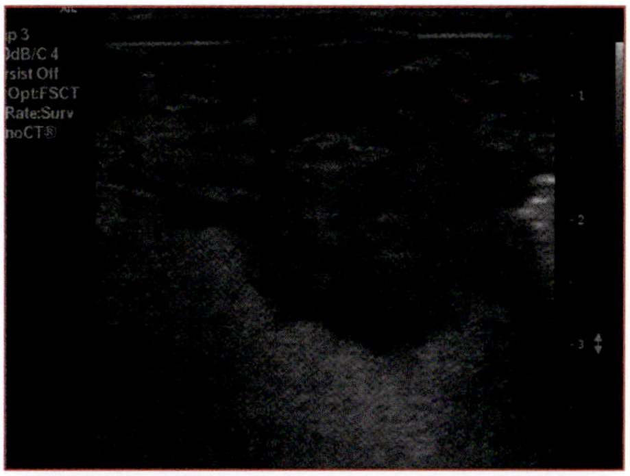

Figure 21. Abdominal ultrasound of a dog with pancreatitis. The right lobe of the pancreas is hypoechoic and the peripancreatic fat appears hyperechoic.

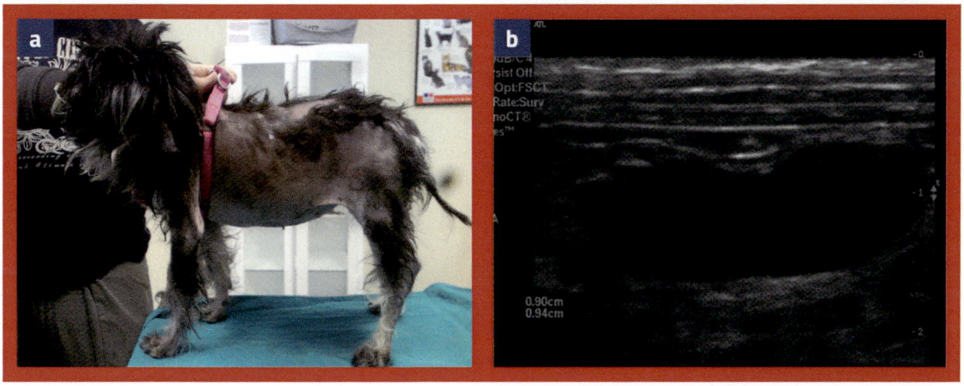

Figure 22. Dog with hyperadrenocorticism (a) and abdominal ultrasound showing enlarged adrenal glands (b).

Diagnostic tests

Diagnostic tests in this type of disorder affecting both the kidneys and the heart will be aimed at diagnosing the primary cause of the damage in both systems, and should also include the tests previously described for evaluating and characterising renal and cardiac dysfunction.

Treatment

Therapeutic management of this condition will target:

- Treating the cause of damage to the cardiovascular and renal system.
- Maintaining haemodynamic stability and ensuring tissue perfusion by the administration of fluid therapy, though this should be done with special care to avoid causing volume overload.
- Controlling cardiovascular complications with the administration of vasopressors and inotropes to maintain filling pressures.
- Acting on renal function by administering fluids to maintain renal perfusion pressure, removing drugs that are potentially nephrotoxic and, where necessary, using dialysis.

03

RENAL DISORDERS SECONDARY TO CARDIOVASCULAR DISEASE

ACUTE CARDIOVASCULAR DISORDERS CAUSING ACUTE KIDNEY INJURY

Alicia Caro Vadillo

CHRONIC CARDIOVASCULAR DISORDERS LEADING TO CHRONIC KIDNEY DISEASE

Javier Duque Carrasco • Rafael Barrera Chacón

ACUTE CARDIOVASCULAR DISORDERS CAUSING ACUTE KIDNEY INJURY

Introduction

There is a very complex – more complex than previously thought – interrelationship between the renal and cardiovascular systems in both healthy and sick individuals. This interaction is the subject of increasing study in all areas: pathogenesis, clinical signs, pathology and treatment, and has led to the concept of cardiorenal syndrome (CRS), also called cardiovascular–renal disorders (CvRD) according to the consensus of the American College of Veterinary Internal Medicine (ACVIM, 2015).

The study of this syndrome has many unresolved uncertainties, but it is clear that there are interactions between these two systems and that blood volume, haemodynamic stability and vasomotor tone of each individual depend on the functionality of both systems.

Within this complex syndrome, five types are described. Type 1 refers to an acute worsening of cardiac function resulting in acute renal impairment.

Aetiology

Acute heart failure is when a rapid onset of clinical signs occurs. It is usually caused by ischaemic processes, but also by worsening of nonischaemic conditions such as valvular diseases or pulmonary embolic conditions, or even by exacerbation of a chronic heart condition refractory to treatment. All these situations require patient hospitalisation. The clinical presentation may range from pulmonary oedema to hypertensive crises or cardiogenic shock. In any of these cases, the kidney responds similarly, by retaining sodium and water.

Acute kidney disease results from a sudden-onset parenchymal kidney injury that leads to generalised failure of the kidneys, which are unable to maintain the body's excretory, metabolic and endocrine demands. This inability results in accumulation of metabolic toxins and disturbances in fluid, electrolyte and acid–base balance.

Pathophysiology

An **acute reduction in cardiac output** causes a decrease in glomerular filtration rate, an increase in creatinine and urea levels in circulating blood, and a decrease in urine production. According to the International Renal Interest Society (IRIS), increases in creatinine of as low as 0.3 mg/dl may be indicative of acute kidney injury and result in a worse prognosis. However, it is not known whether these changes indicate permanent structural damage to the kidney itself. The therapeutic recommendation is to treat patients with acute heart failure with the lowest dose of diuretics capable of controlling congestive signs. This makes it essential to monitor creatinine levels continuously in patients with acute heart failure.

Other mechanisms in addition to decreased cardiac output have been proposed as leading to kidney injury, such as **renal congestion** due to increased venous pressure. This increase in venous pressure causes an increase in capsular pressure, thus decreasing the gradient between such capsular hydrostatic pressure and glomerular blood pressure, which leads to a decreased glomerular filtration gradient and a fall in renal function.

One of the main objectives of the treatment of heart failure is the control of venous congestion, while taking into account the negative effect of diuretic drugs on renal arterial perfusion and not only their positive effect on renal venous congestion.

On the other hand, activation of the renin–angiotensin–aldosterone system (RAAS), with subsequent release of **angiotensin II,** will induce oxidation- and cytokine-mediated lesions, inflammation and cell death, leading to endothelial dysfunction and formation of oxidative substances that contribute to renal injury and cardiac dysfunction.

Pathophysiology of acute heart failure

Acute heart failure (AHF) is defined as the onset of clinical signs of heart impairment or rapid worsening of pre-existing heart failure requiring urgent treatment. The development of AHF involves several pathophysiological mechanisms and factors that trigger circulatory decompensation.

From a pathophysiological viewpoint, heart dysfunction (including acute myocardial damage and remodelling) occurs in AHF together with dysfunction of systemic and pulmonary circulation that also includes endothelial dysfunction. This cardiac and endothelial dysfunction leads to severe acute haemodynamic disturbances. Factors triggering AHF include myocardial ischaemia, systemic arterial hypertension, arrhythmias, other concomitant non-cardiac diseases, and drugs administered, among others.

AHF is characterised by the presence of three phenomena:

1. **Neurohormonal activation:** includes activation of the RAAS, sympathetic nervous system, arginine–vasopressin axis, endothelin, adrenomedullin, and natriuretic peptide system.
2. **Inflammatory activation:** includes activation of the innate immune response, increased expression of proinflammatory mediators such as tumour necrosis factor (TNF), interleukin-1 (IL-1), interleukin-6 (IL-6), etc., among other inflammatory responses.
3. **Oxidative stress:** it is associated with an excess of reactive oxygen species that alter physiology and lead to the production of toxic substances.

Haemodynamic response

AHF is associated with various abnormal haemodynamic responses, including a significant reduction in cardiac output, increased filling pressures, and increased afterload.

As AHF may include a wide range of clinical abnormalities with different pathophysiology and different triggering factors, patients with AHF may present with different clinical signs.

The initial clinical diagnosis of AHF is based on the presence of compatible clinical signs and is confirmed by diagnostic tests such as electrocardiograms, chest X-rays, blood tests including measurement of biomarkers such as troponins, and echocardiography. Clinical signs are most commonly secondary to pulmonary oedema (Fig. 1), but there may be cases related to an acute reduction in cardiac output, as may occur in severe arrhythmia (Figs. 2–5). Other situations involving the sudden onset of low cardiac output may include rupture of the chordae tendineae in patients with chronic mitral valve degeneration, acute pericardial effusions due to bleeding masses, decompensations of chronic conditions, and severe acute systolic dysfunction, as may occur in infectious or other myocardial conditions (Figs. 6–10).

Physical examination of patients suspected of having AHF is important and should include blood pressure, temperature, presence/absence of jugular venous distension or jugular pulse, hepatomegaly, ascites, peripheral oedema, and determination of the level of consciousness. In a hospital setting, urine output should be monitored.

One of the main signs of AHF is the presence of pulmonary oedema. In human medicine and for many clinicians, **pulmonary oedema** is the real clinical presentation of AHF with a sudden onset of typical clinical signs such as tachypnoea and resting orthopnoea (Fig. 11).

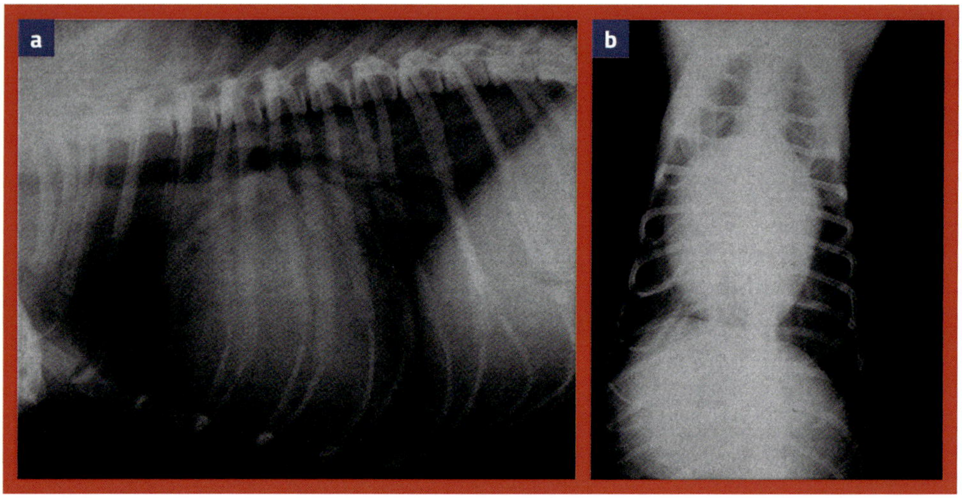

Figure 1. Right lateral (a) and ventrodorsal (b) X-rays of a patient with cardiomegaly and a vascular and interstitial pattern consistent with lung oedema in a dog. Images courtesy of the Diagnostic Imaging Department of Complutense Veterinary Teaching Hospital.

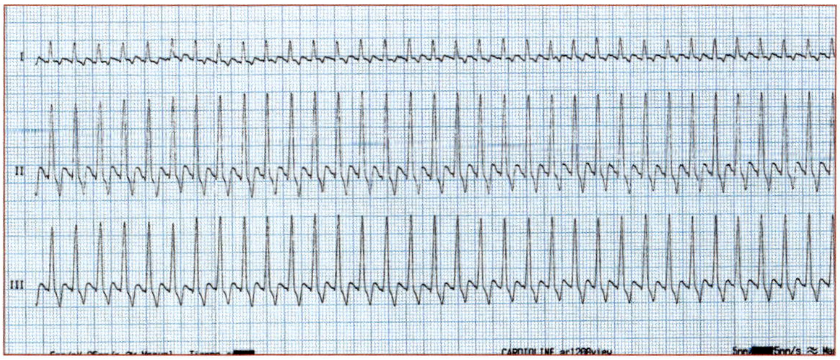

Figure 2. ECG in leads I, II and III in a patient with supraventricular tachycardia at a rate of 300 bpm, causing a low cardiac output.

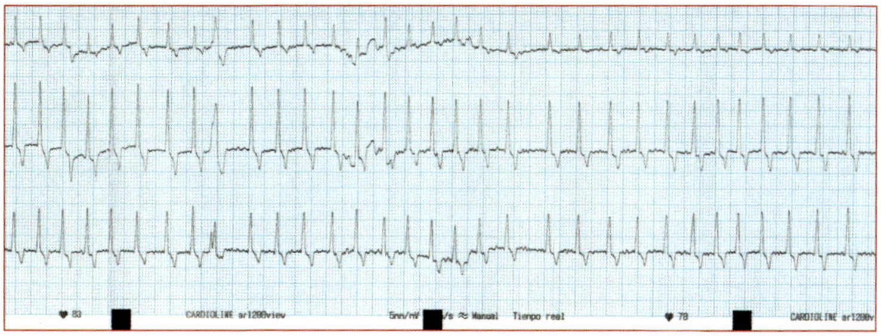

Figure 3. ECG in leads I, II and III in a patient with atrial fibrillation and right ventricular premature complex.

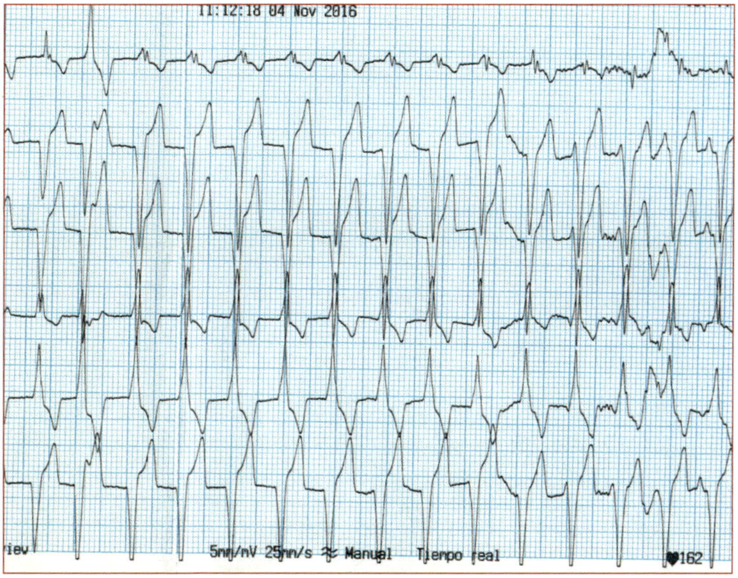

Figure 4. Six-lead ECG in a patient with multifocal ventricular tachycardia. The second complex shows a different morphology in lead I as compared to the rest.

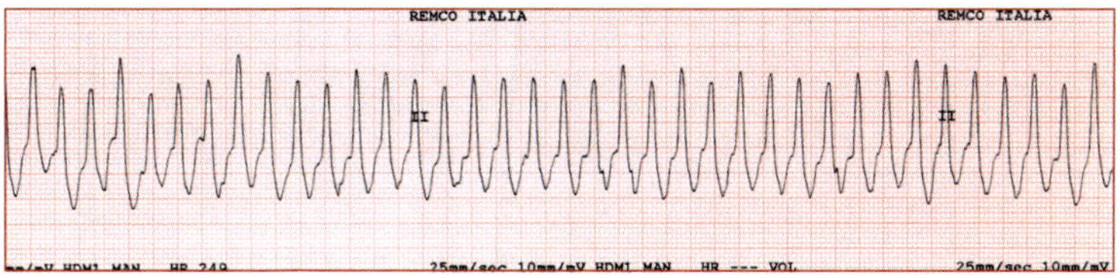

Figure 5. ECG in lead II of a patient with continuous right ventricular tachycardia at a rate higher than 300 bpm.

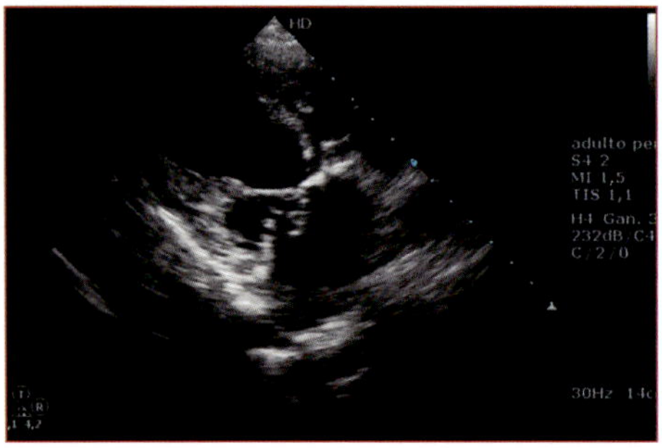

Figure 6. Echocardiography. Right parasternal long-axis four-chamber view in a patient with chordae tendineae rupture, probably secondary to chronic mitral valve disease.

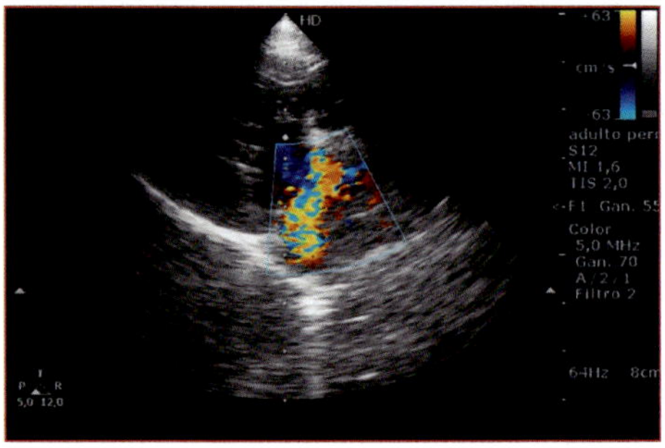

Figure 7. Echocardiography. Right parasternal long-axis four-chamber view of the same patient from the above figure showing mitral regurgitation flow.

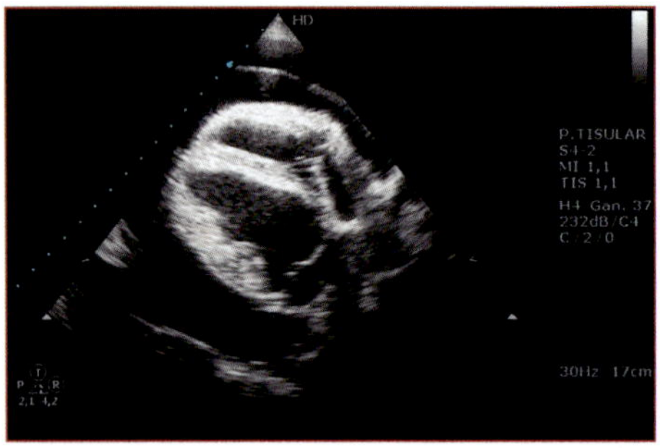

Figure 8. Echocardiography. Right parasternal long-axis four-chamber view in a patient with pericardial effusion, cardiac tamponade, and pleural effusion. Cardiac tamponade shows low cardiac output and hypotension.

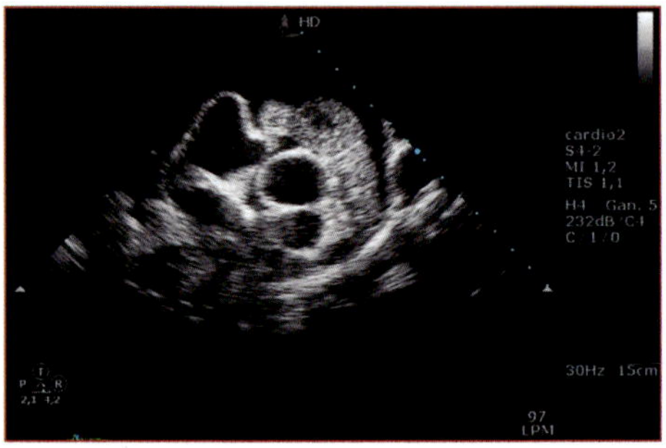

Figure 9. Echocardiography. Right parasternal short-axis view of the aorta in a patient with pericardial effusion, cardiac tamponade, and pleural effusion. Cardiac tamponade shows low cardiac output and hypotension.

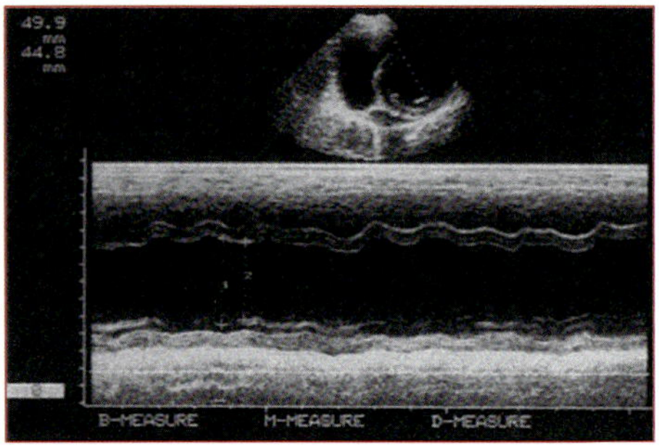

Figure 10. M-mode echocardiography in a patient with severe systolic dysfunction.

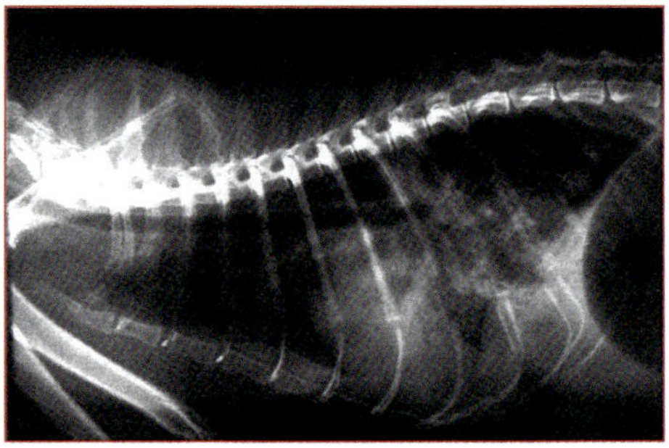

Figure 11. Right lateral X-ray of a feline patient with pulmonary oedema of cardiogenic origin. Image courtesy of the Diagnostic Imaging Department of Complutense Veterinary Teaching Hospital.

In other cases, AHF appears as a **hypertensive crisis**. It is associated with elevated systemic blood pressure and accompanied by respiratory signs. These patients show no clear clinical signs of pulmonary oedema, but dyspnoea and tachypnoea are found, and vasoconstriction is the predominant reason for this clinical picture (Fig. 12).

This is important when establishing different treatment strategies, since some patients will require more diuretic treatment and others a combination of vasodilating drugs and diuretics.

Heart failure sometimes arises from cardiogenic shock, characterised by severe peripheral hypoperfusion and lesions in different organs due to low systemic blood pressures and low urine output.

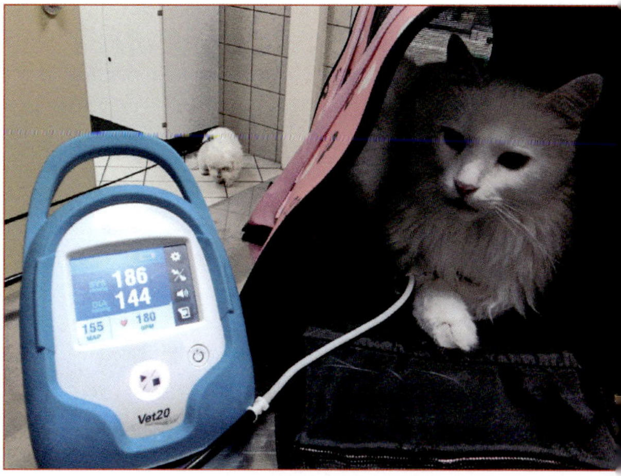

Figure 12. Feline patient with systemic hypertension.

Worsening renal function

Acute kidney injury (AKI) in patients with AHF is basically defined as an increase in serum creatinine levels by more than 0.3 mg/dl during a period of hospitalisation due to AHF.

The IRIS has proposed diagnostic criteria for AKI in dogs and cats (Table 1). AKI may result from prerenal and postrenal changes, but we will limit our discussion to prerenal conditions as the focus of this section is CvRD type 1.

It is important to remember that the use of drugs such as angiotensin-converting enzyme inhibitors (ACEIs), widely generalised in all cases of both acute and chronic heart failure, can cause nephrotoxicity at high doses or when administered to hypovolaemic patients. Similarly, treatment with high-ceiling diuretic drugs at high doses is associated with decreased blood volume and worsening renal function.

Table 1. IRIS classification of acute kidney injury (AKI).

AKI grade	Creatinine	Clinical signs
Grade I	<1.6 mg/dl	■ No azotaemia. ■ Evidence of oliguria or anuria ■ Creatinine levels increase by >0.3 mg/dl in the last 48 hours.
Grade II	1.7–2.5 mg/dl	Mild AKI.
Grade III	2.6-5 mg/dl	Moderate to severe AKI.
Grade IV	5.1–10 mg/dl	
Grade V	>10 mg/dl	

Haemodynamic mechanisms

There is a range of evidence that haemodynamic function plays an important role in the pathophysiology of CvRD type 1.

- **Low cardiac output and renal hypoperfusion.** Decreased cardiac output leads to decreased renal perfusion. Compensatory mechanisms such as sympathetic nervous system and RAAS stimulation as well as vasopressin secretion result in enhanced sodium and water reabsorption to preserve renal perfusion and glomerular filtration. These long-term actions lead to negative effects on the heart and kidney, causing fibrosis, apoptosis and ventricular remodelling. Additionally, constant hypoperfusion leads to ischaemia of the cortical parenchyma that further affects kidney function.
- **Fluid overload and renal venous congestion.** Elevated central venous pressure (CVP) has been shown to reduce renal blood flow and glomerular filtration rate. Congestion of the kidneys increases capsular pressure, decreases glomerular filtration pressure, and significantly decreases renal function. Increased pressure in renal veins also induces an increase in interstitial pressure, leading to tubular compression, hypoxia, and a greater decrease in glomerular filtration rate. In addition, external compression of the parenchyma and renal veins due to increased abdominal pressure also worsens renal function.

Neurohormonal mechanisms

The RAAS and the sympathetic nervous system are involved in worsening renal function:

- **RAAS.** In acute hypoperfusion conditions, the RAAS maintains glomerular filtration, but its chronic stimulation causes cell hypertrophy, fibrosis, oxidative stress, and activation of inflammation.
- **Sympathetic nervous system.** Increases vascular tone and also predisposes to apoptosis and fibrosis.

Inflammatory mechanisms

Increases in cytokine levels, including tumour necrosis factor α and other markers of inflammation, have been reported during the development of heart failure. This high concentration of cytokines reduces iron absorption and also reduces the action of angiotensin-converting enzyme. Since angiotensin II is a substance that promotes erythropoietin secretion, these higher cytokine levels contribute to the anaemia described in humans. Low levels of erythropoietin reduce haemoglobin levels. In addition, as levels of erythropoietin decrease, so do its antioxidant properties, which leads to increased oxidative stress and contributes to the development of CvRD.

Intrinsic tubular lesions

Decreased perfusion and ischaemia are important factors in the development of tubular lesions in the course of AHF. In fact, some markers of tubular damage, such as neutrophil gelatinase-associated lipocalin (NGAL), are elevated in urine and plasma long before creatinine increases in patients with AHF (Fig. 13).

Diagnosis

Urea and creatinine

They are the most classic indicators of renal function, but their values are influenced by muscle mass, RAAS activation and vasopressin, among other factors. Diagnosis of AKI is challenging due to the lack of early biomarkers. In fact, when urea and creatinine levels are elevated, the renal injury process is already very well established. The ideal marker of AKI secondary to AHF should be sensitive and specific for renal injury, with no external influences, and should serve as a guide for treatments.

New markers

Several molecules detectable in blood or urine are being studied:

- Glomerular damage. Cystatin C is a protein that is filtered by glomeruli but is not secreted and is independent of muscle mass, protein consumption, etc. The concentration of this protein in urine reflects kidney-specific functions.
- Tubular damage. Neutrophil gelatinase-associated lipocalin (NGAL), kidney injury molecule-1 (KIM-1) and N-acetyl-β-D-glucosaminidase are new proposed markers for diagnosis of AKI secondary to AHF. There are no veterinary studies in this same context (AHF + AKI), except for NGAL.
- Glomerular filtration rate. Symmetric dimethylarginine (SDMA) has been evaluated in human medicine as a negative prognostic factor for AHF. No veterinary studies are available yet for cases of AHF, but it has shown its value in chronic heart failure situations.

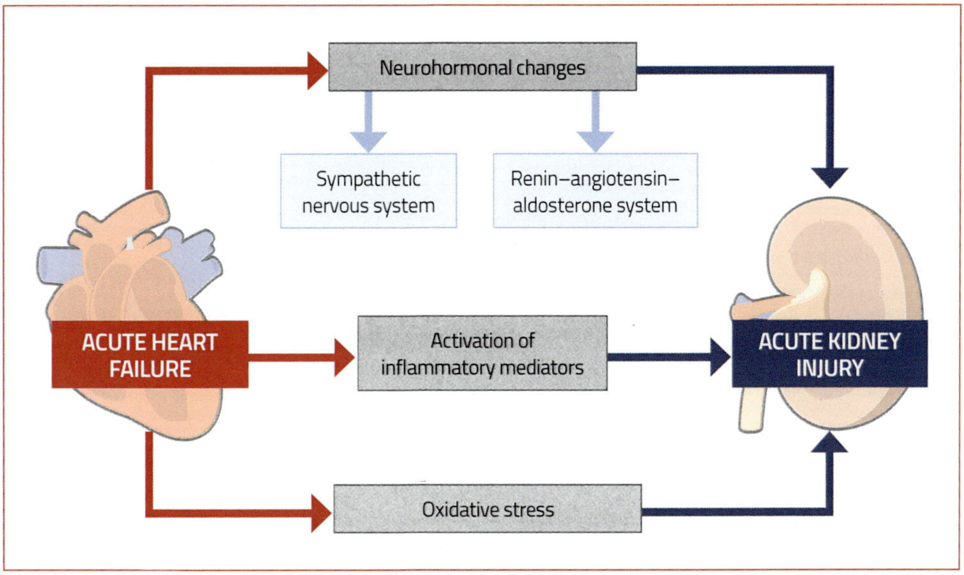

Figure 13. Diagram of the self-perpetuating relationship between acute heart failure and acute kidney injury.

Clinical management

As studies of CvRDs in animals are scarce, the proposed treatments are based on experiences and not on medical scientific evidence. This makes it likely that the following recommendations will change as more evidence emerges.

Treatment is based on the use of diuretics; the most indicated are high-dose loop diuretics for short periods of time, without forgetting the need for subsequent titration.

Aggressive decongestion increases renal and myocardial flow and improves ventricular preload conditions. These facts allow renal function to improve sufficiently to maintain urine output with lower doses of diuretics. The lowest dose of diuretic required to resolve congestive signs should be administered, and renal function should be assessed at all times.

There are two predictors of poor renal tolerance to acute diuresis: heart failure due to new onset diastolic failure and the lack of peripheral oedema. Diuresis in the absence of peripheral oedema will cause significant changes in cardiac output and, therefore, renal injury and hypotension. In these cases treatment will depend more on vasodilating drugs.

The clinical response of AHF patients to diuretic therapy is highly variable and depends on the balance between adequate renal perfusion and minimal venous congestion. An excess in the diuretic effect causes a reduction in intravascular volume and, therefore, a reduction in renal perfusion with impairment of its function. In contrast, a decrease in venous congestion would improve glomerular filtration. Thus, it has been suggested that high-dose diuretics are beneficial in acute volume overload conditions, but these doses are harmful in patients with minimal volume overload.

Treatments based on inodilator drugs and neurohormonal antagonists that could be helpful in patients with hypertensive crises and AHF have also been proposed.

Other alternatives used to reduce worsening of renal function include ultrafiltration, vasopressin inhibitors, natriuretic peptides, and pimobendan, but little data is available on their efficacy in veterinary practice.

CHRONIC CARDIOVASCULAR DISORDERS LEADING TO CHRONIC KIDNEY DISEASE

Introduction

In 2015, a consensus group formed by veterinary specialists (Pouchelon et al., 2015) defined the cardiorenal syndrome described in human medicine (Ronco et al., 2008), renaming it for dogs and cats as **cardiovascular–renal disorders** (CvRD). This chapter will discuss the primary disorders that chronically affect the cardiovascular system and that will have a secondary impact on renal function ($CvRD_{CH}$). The most common causes leading to this situation are those described next.

Aetiology

Heart diseases affecting dogs and cats that have been studied in the context of $CvRD_{CH}$ include mitral valve degeneration, dilated cardiomyopathy, and hypertrophic cardiomyopathy in cats.

Mitral valve degeneration

Mitral valve degeneration (MVD) (Fig. 1) is the most common acquired heart disease in dogs. Decreased cardiac output as well as haemodynamic changes resulting from activation of neurohormonal systems may affect renal function, leading to a decrease in glomerular filtration rate (GFR) (Chetboul et al., 2012).

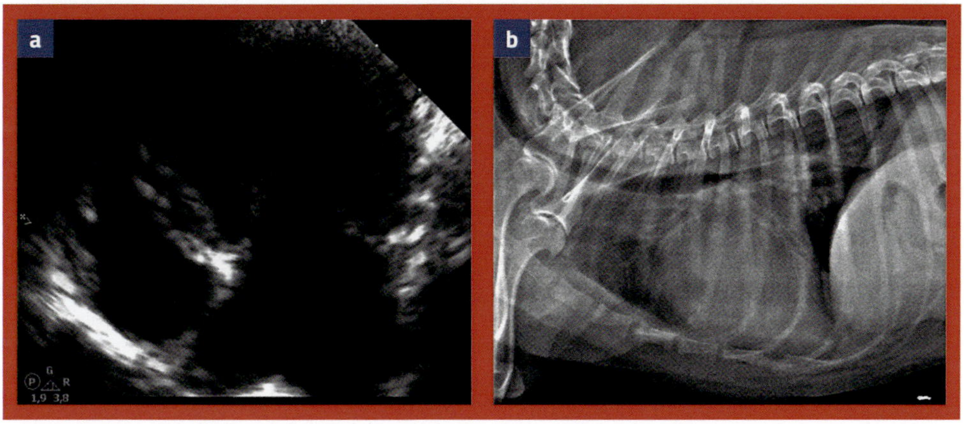

Figure 1. Echocardiography showing a left apical section in a dog with mitral valve degeneration. Left atrial enlargement as well as mitral valve thickening are seen (a). Lateral chest X-ray of the same dog showing signs of cardiomegaly with evident enlargement of the left atrium (b).

In a study of 124 dogs with this heart disease (Nicolle et al., 2007), 50 % were azotaemic and up to 70 % of patients had azotaemia in the later stages of the disease, so one of the most relevant conclusions drawn from this study was that the prevalence of azotaemia increased with the severity of heart failure (HF). This could be explained mainly by the effect of heart disease on renal function, the action of drugs administered in the advanced stages of heart disease (79 %, 63 % and 4 % of dogs with MVD classified as New York Heart Association [NYHA] class 4 were treated with furosemide, ACEIs, and digoxin, respectively), and the effect of age and concomitant chronic kidney disease (CKD).

Dilated cardiomyopathy

Few studies have been conducted on the interaction between chronic HF due to dilated cardiomyopathy (DCM) (Fig. 2), CKD and anaemia as a vicious cycle in dogs. The interaction between these three conditions causes a deterioration in cardiac and renal function and leads to a worsening of anaemia. In a study comparing a group of healthy dogs with another group of dogs with DCM, significant differences were found in red blood cells, haemoglobin and haematocrit (Srivastava et al., 2015). Both anaemia and kidney disease are associated with an increased activation of mechanisms that play an important role in disease progression.

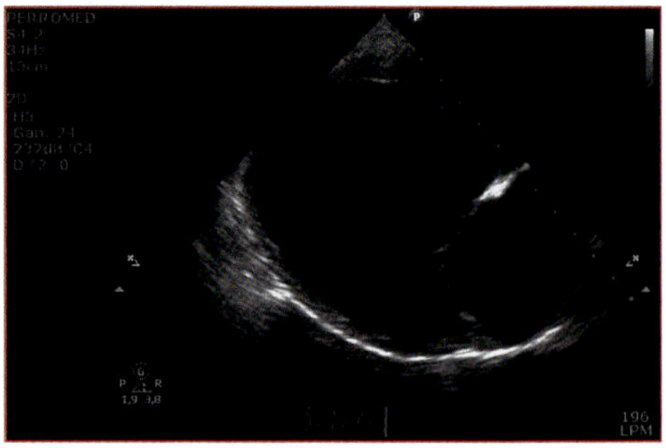

Figure 2. Echocardiography of a dog with dilated cardiomyopathy in a right parasternal long-axis view, where a large dilation of both the left ventricle and left atrium can be seen.

Hypertrophic cardiomyopathy in cats

In advanced stages of hypertrophic cardiomyopathy (HCM) (Fig. 3), stroke volume is decreased, which significantly compromises perfusion of vital organs such as the kidneys. During the course of this heart disease (the most common in cats), renal hypoperfusion, activation of the sympathetic nervous system and increased activity of the renin–angiotensin–aldosterone system (RAAS) may occur, and lead to different degrees of secondary renal dysfunction. In a retrospective study including 102 cats with HCM (Gouni et al., 2008), 59 % were found to have azotaemia. Although this percentage was higher than in the control group, the statistical study showed no significant differences between both groups. When patients with this cardiomyopathy were assessed, no differences were seen either between those with or without congestive heart failure, so in contrast to what has been reported in dogs with mitral valve degeneration, the severity of cardiac disease has not been shown to be related to the degree of azotaemia in cats.

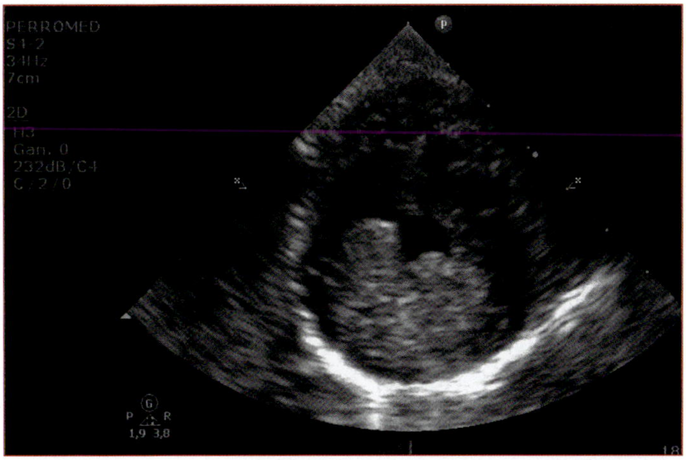

Figure 3. Left ventricular echocardiography in the short axis of a cat with hypertrophic cardiomyopathy.

Other causes described in the guidelines proposed in 2015 by the consensus group for $CVRD_{CH}$ are:

- Congestion of the kidneys during heart failure (Fig. 4).
- Filariosis or vena cava syndrome leading to the development of glomerular disease (Fig. 5).

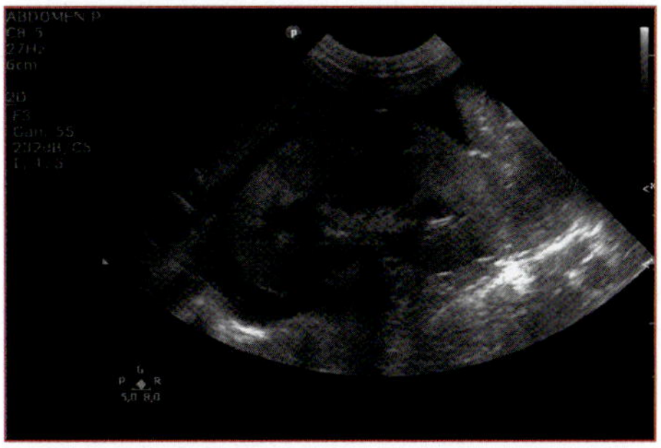

Figure 4. Abdominal ultrasound showing a kidney surrounded by free fluid in a dog with ascites due to right congestive heart failure.

Pathophysiology

$CvRD_{CH}$ refers to renal dysfunction or damage occurring as a result of a primary disease affecting the cardiovascular system. Potential pathophysiological mechanisms leading to $CvRD_{CH}$ include decreased renal perfusion secondary to decreased cardiac output, activation of neuroendocrine systems such as the RAAS and the sympathetic nervous system, generation of reactive oxygen species due to endothelial damage and venous congestion of the kidneys (Vaden et al., 2017).

In both humans and animals, decreased cardiac output may result in decreased GFR with an increase in urea and creatinine levels, and if this situation persists over time, structural damage may occur in the kidneys that may lead to a poorer prognosis.

Patients with heart disease receive diuretics as part of therapy to resolve signs of congestion. This will result in reduced intravascular volume, leading to activation of the RAAS and the sympathetic nervous system and to decreased renal perfusion. All of this will contribute to the development of kidney dysfunction and damage, resulting in $CvRD_{CH}$.

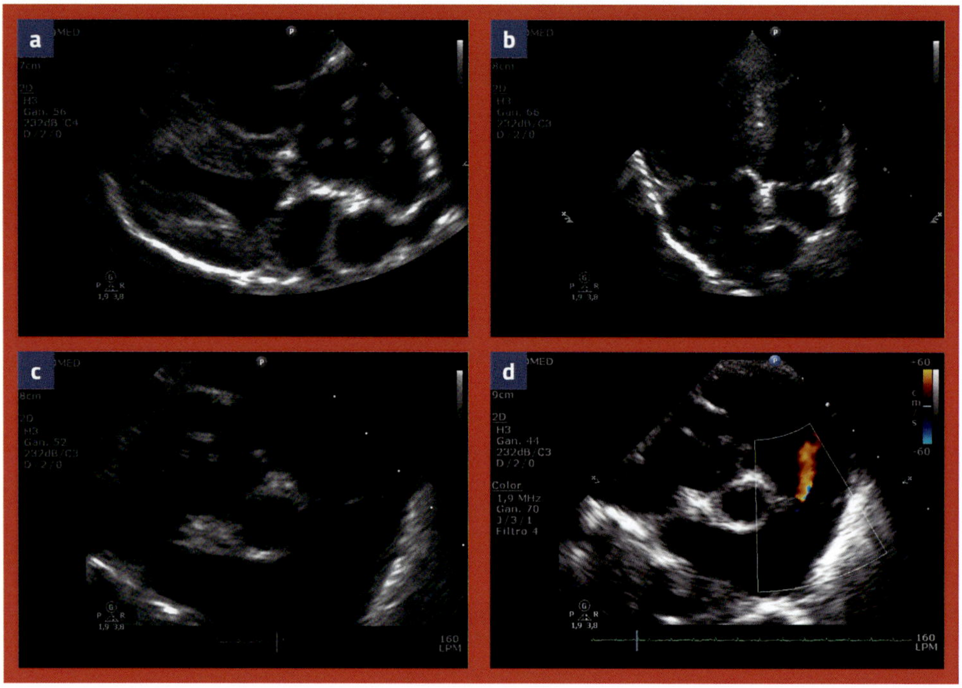

Figure 5. Echocardiography in a dog with filariosis. In the right parasternal four-chamber view (a) and in the left apical view (b), adult *Dirofilaria immitis* worms can be seen in the right atrium, as well as dilation of the right chambers and hypertrophy of the interventricular septum. The cardiac base shows significant dilation of the pulmonary artery (c) and pulmonary regurgitation (d) associated with pulmonary hypertension.

Venous congestion affects haemodynamic regulation of glomerular filtration through activation of mechanisms causing vasoconstriction of the afferent arteriole and thus reduces GFR. Congestion of kidney tissue due to poor heart function and high systemic venous pressure leads to an increase in capsular pressure, a decrease in blood pressure and GFR and, consequently, to a decrease in kidney function. In human medicine, in patients with HF, incomplete resolution of venous congestion is one of the leading causes of impaired renal function and has been associated with a worse prognosis. This situation creates a dilemma when attempting to achieve a balance between the negative effects derived from the use of diuretics on renal perfusion and the positive effects on correcting venous congestion.

The RAAS, and specifically angiotensin II, leads to oxidative damage and damage associated with cytokine release, resulting in cell inflammation and death. Endothelial changes and the formation of reactive oxygen species are an important link between renal and cardiac dysfunction. On the other hand, congestive HF and elevated cytokine levels will result in decreased iron absorption.

In addition, angiotensin-converting enzyme inhibitors, routinely used in patients with HF, lead to decreased erythropoietin production (angiotensin II stimulates erythropoietin secretion). All of this contributes to the development of anaemia in human medicine. However, the role of haemoglobin in $CvRD_{CH}$ development is not yet clear.

Finally, within the definition of $CvRD_{CH}$ are included vascular diseases such as systemic arterial hypertension (SHT), which cause glomerular damage.

Diagnosis

Diagnostic imaging

Diagnostic imaging techniques provide evidence for the presence, cause, severity, and consequences of heart disease.

Radiology

The goal of radiography in heart patients is to detect changes in the size of the cardiac silhouette (Figs. 6 and 7) and vascular structures (Fig. 8), as well as airway and lung parenchymal changes (Fig. 9). These changes are used to confirm the presence of signs consistent with cardiac disease or congestive heart failure.

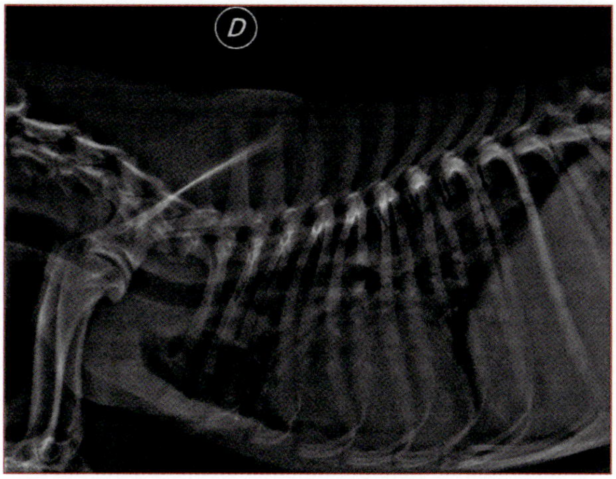

Figure 6. Lateral chest X-rays of a dog with heartworm disease showing enlargement of the cardiac silhouette, particularly due to increased size of right heart chambers.

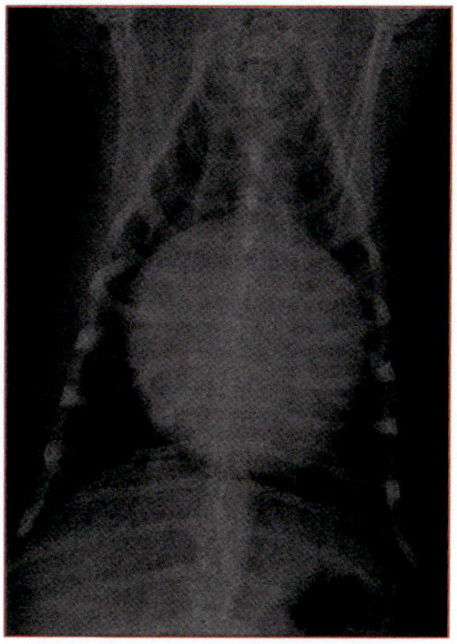

Figure 7. Ventrodorsal chest X-ray showing evident cardiomegaly.

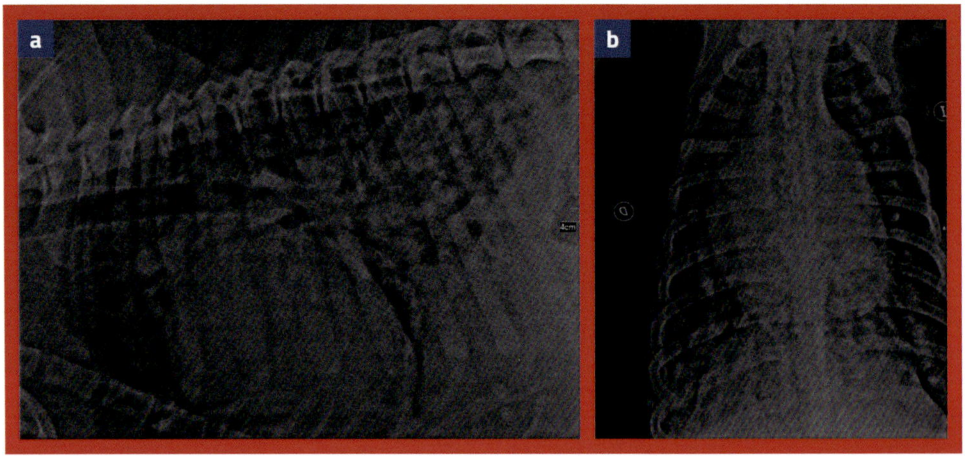

Figure 8. Lateral (a) and ventrodorsal (b) X-rays of a dog with heartworm disease showing a vascular pattern.

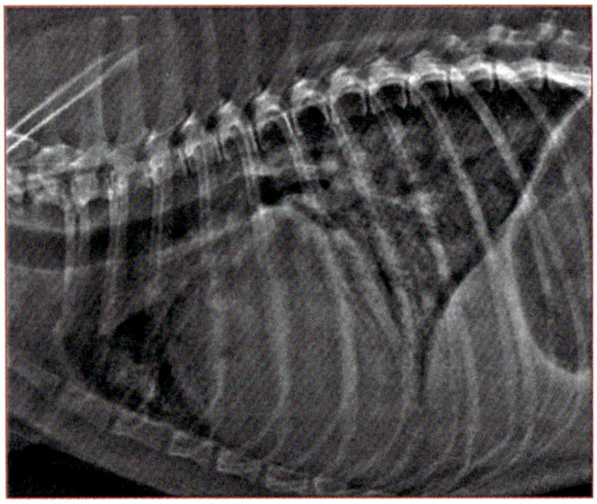

Figure 9. Lateral chest X-ray showing pulmonary oedema in a dog with mitral valve degeneration.

Ultrasound

Ultrasound is useful for detecting changes in both morphology (Fig. 10) and heart function (Fig. 11) in early and advanced stages of the disease. Doppler ultrasound (spectral, pulsed and continuous) (Fig. 12) as well as other more advanced modalities – tissue Doppler, deformation analysis (strain and strain rate imaging) and speckle-tracking – provide information about the direction and speed of blood flow and myocardial function.

Blood pressure measurement

One of the best known interactions between the cardiovascular system and the kidneys is the fact that both organs are involved in blood pressure regulation, so measurement of blood pressure is recommended as a routine test in patients with kidney or heart disease.

In both dogs and cats, SHT is a potential cause of irreversible damage to the heart and kidneys. In dogs, SHT has been associated with a decrease in GFR, as well as an increase in kidney damage, proteinuria, uraemic crises, and death. In cats, the relationship between SHT and kidney disease, however, is not so clear. Increased blood pressure has been shown to be a risk factor for proteinuria, which in turn leads to worsening of kidney disease.

The consequences of SHT on the cardiovascular system include development of left ventricular hypertrophy, arrhythmias, bleeding, myocardial remodelling and fibrosis, aortic insufficiency, diastolic dysfunction, and HF.

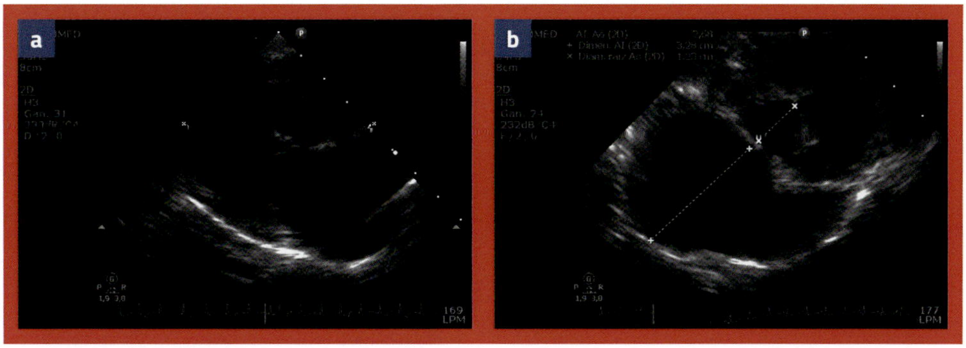

Figure 10. Echocardiography of a dog with mitral valve degeneration showing thickening of the mitral valve in the right parasternal long-axis view (a) and left atrial enlargement when compared to aortic diameter (b).

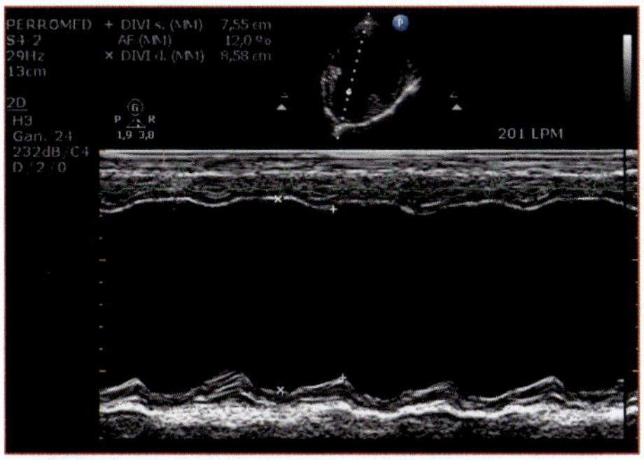

Figure 11. M-mode echocardiography of a dog with dilated cardiomyopathy showing left ventricular dilation and a low shortening fraction.

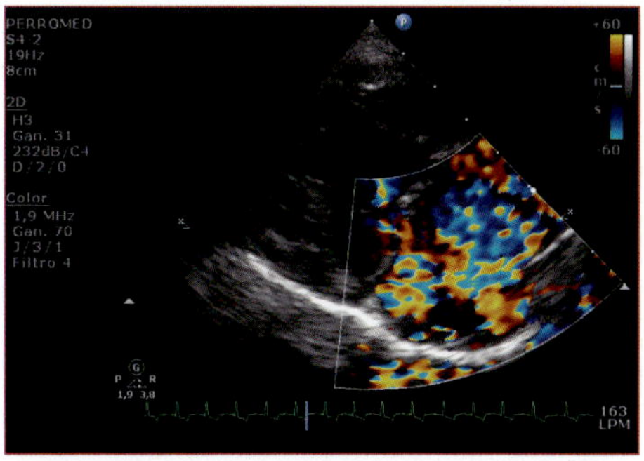

Figure 12. Echocardiography of a dog with mitral valve degeneration in which colour Doppler shows mitral regurgitation.

For a greater understanding of the diagnosis and treatment of SHT in dogs and cats, the authors recommend reading the *ACVIM consensus statement: Guidelines for the identification, evaluation, and management of systemic hypertension in dogs and cats* (Acierno et al., 2018).

Laboratory tests

Biomarkers are substances made by a tissue that can be detected in the bloodstream by laboratory testing. As requirements, they must be released in an amount proportional to the course of the disease, provide information on the presence, severity and prognosis of the disease, be stable and easy to determine through tests that are available to any clinician, be fast and economical to perform. In this regard, biomarkers of kidney disease and heart disease are available for $CvRD_{CH}$ assessment (Fig. 13).

Kidney disease biomarkers

Renal function parameters that have been studied in the context of $CvRD_{CH}$ are those described next.

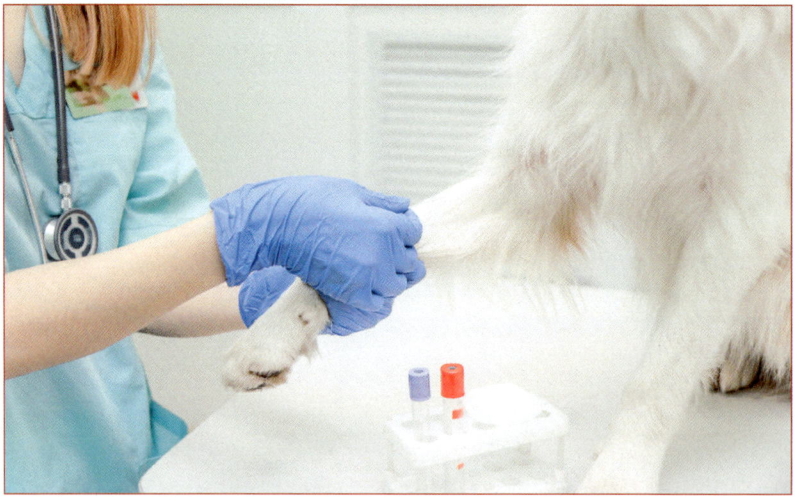

Figure 13. Blood sampling in a canine patient (Ermolaev Alexander, Shutterstock.com).

Urea and creatinine

In 2016, a study in 158 dogs with chronic MVD showed that 25 % of patients had azotaemia (Martinelli et al., 2016). This increase in urea and creatinine may be due to the decrease in renal perfusion associated with the course of heart disease, as well as the administration of drugs such as diuretics (Boswood and Murphy, 2005; Martinelli et al., 2016; Nicolle et al., 2007). In addition, the presence of renal disease in patients with MVD was found to be associated with a decrease in survival time, so early diagnosis of renal dysfunction in patients with cardiovascular disease is of vital importance. However, the data obtained from studies conducted in cats with HCM differ from the results obtained in dogs. Thus, in a population of 102 HCM cats, 59 % of them with azotaemia (Gouni et al., 2008), there was no relationship between urea and creatinine values and echocardiographic variables, and no clear association was found between heart disease severity and azotaemia.

GFR is considered the best parameter to quantify renal filtration; however, it is not routinely measured in dogs or cats, since it requires intravenous administration of a filtration marker followed by multiple blood samplings in a given time, which is impractical.

Diagnosis of CKD is currently based on measurement of plasma creatinine, among other biomarkers. Plasma creatinine is the most commonly used indicator for assessing GFR. However, the main disadvantage of evaluation of this parameter is that the increase in plasma creatinine occurs when 75 % of kidney function has been lost. It is therefore necessary to search for new biomarkers that allow early detection of renal dysfunction in the $CvRD_{CH}$ scenario. In this regard, the markers described next have been studied.

Cystatin C

It has a significant advantage over other biomarkers, such as creatinine, as it detects renal failure earlier.

In a study of 33 dogs with MVD (Choi et al., 2016) and which were divided into the different groups proposed by the International Small Animal Cardiac Health Council (ISACHC), cystatin C was found to be able to show renal dysfunction before creatinine. This would allow detection of decreased GFR in the early stages of heart disease, which would make it possible for the veterinary clinician to intervene early, even in asymptomatic cardiac patients, and successfully treat HF in dogs with chronic valve degeneration in the long term.

Symmetric dimethylarginine

An increase in symmetric dimethylarginine (SDMA) in plasma can be detected before one in creatinine and it can identify a 30 % decrease in GFR.

In the few studies where the value of SDMA in dogs with heart disease has been determined (Choi et al., 2016; Savarese et al., 2018), specifically in patients with MVD, it has been found to be a useful laboratory parameter for assessing renal function in dogs with this valvular disease, particularly in less advanced stages (ACVIM B2), in which an early diagnosis of renal dysfunction is very important in relation to the use of diuretics as part of the therapeutic plan.

In cats, however, the results are not consistent with those observed in dogs. A study of the value of SDMA in 40 cats with HCM (Langhorn et al., 2018) showed that this heart disease did not affect the level of this renal dysfunction biomarker.

Neutrophil gelatinase-associated lipocalin

Neutrophil gelatinase-associated lipocalin (NGAL) has been found to increase earlier than creatinine in animals with kidney disease. Its increase suggests tubular damage, and since the tubule is sensitive to a decrease in renal perfusion and hypoxic damage as a result of HF, the tubule may be damaged while the renal cortex is intact, maintaining GFR. On the other hand, renal blood flow can fall between 30 % and 40 % without apparently affecting GFR. All of these factors make tubular damage biomarkers such as NGAL more sensitive than creatinine.

Thus, in a study conducted on 31 dogs with HF due to MVD (Jung et al., 2018), it was suggested that the presence of $CvRD_{CH}$, undetectable with routine tests in dogs with HF, could be predicted with the detection of elevations in NGAL values at the time of patient admission.

Cardiac disease biomarkers

N-terminal pro–B-type natriuretic peptide and cardiac troponin I

The specific parameters evaluated in cardiac diseases are usually N-terminal pro–B-type natriuretic peptide (NT-proBNP) and cardiac troponin I (cTnI). Natriuretic peptides are produced by the myocardium and help regulate plasma volume, sodium excretion, and vascular tone in both healthy and diseased animals. Some studies have also been conducted (Oyama, 2013) in which cTnI and NT-proBNP were measured in dogs with kidney disease and found to have increased values, probably because their excretion is urinary and is decreased in case of renal dysfunction. Because of this, in the setting of kidney disease, it is difficult to determine whether the increase in these biomarkers is due to heart disease or to a decrease in renal clearance.

Haematology

Although in human medicine the study of anaemia in the setting of $CvRD_{CH}$ has raised interest to the point of speaking of a cardiorenal anaemia syndrome, few studies on this aspect have been conducted in veterinary medicine.

Anaemia in dogs affected by heart disease may be due to decreased erythropoietin synthesis as a result of CKD. Other important factors in the development of anaemia are haemolysis associated with elevated urea levels in kidney disease and tumour necrosis factor in heart disease.

Correction of anaemia does not replace treatment for HF, but appears to be important for improving cardiac muscle function, and both anaemia and renal dysfunction have been shown to be associated with increased mortality in human patients with congestive HF. In dogs, the presence of anaemia has also been shown to predict a poorer prognosis in patients with MVD (Yu and Huang, 2016). However, no studies have yet shown that correction of anaemia improves prognosis in dogs with this valvular disease.

Clinical management

It is a challenge for the veterinary surgeon for several reasons, one of which is the fact that animals with HF require the administration of diuretics to fight congestion. On the one hand, there is a tendency for patients receiving diuretics to develop azotaemia and, on the other hand, a tendency for patients receiving fluid therapy to develop congestion, which greatly complicates $CvRD_{CH}$ management (Fig. 14).

In this regard, the therapeutic window for this condition is small, as both the use of diuretics and ACE inhibitors (ACEIs) can cause adverse effects on renal function (Atkins et al., 2002).

HF occurs when the heart fails to provide adequate cardiac output or is only able to ensure it with high filling venous pressures and a risk of congestion. Treatment of chronic HF involves the use of:

- Diuretics such as furosemide
- Vasodilators such as ACEIs, amlodipine, nitroglycerin, and nitroprusside
- Neurohormonal activation blocking agents such as ACEIs, spironolactone, and beta-blockers
- Positive inotropes such as digoxin, dobutamine, and pimobendan

In the case of congestive heart failure, excessive vascular volume reduction can lead to adverse effects on the kidneys. In this regard, achieving a balance in therapy is exponentially more difficult when the heart and kidneys suffer dysfunction concomitantly. Treatment of $CvRD_{CH}$ involves simultaneous recognition and evaluation of subtle changes in cardiac and renal function and understanding of how the pathophysiology of one of the conditions interacts and influences the function of the other organ. An important point in the management of $CvRD_{CH}$ is to treat the clinical signs of the primary cause to minimise worsening of the other system.

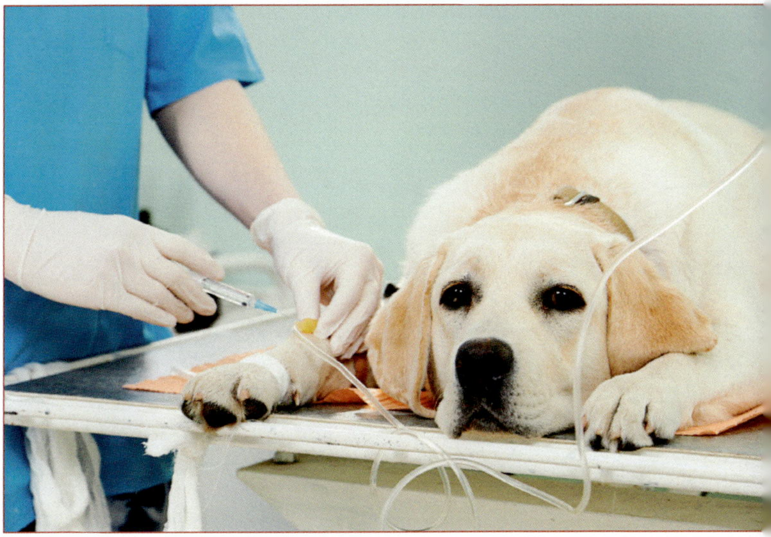

Figure 14. Achieving a balance in diuretic therapy and fluid intake is crucial for $CvRD_{CH}$ management (Dmitry Kalinovsky, Shutterstock.com).

Unfortunately, for now, $CvRD_{CH}$ treatment guidelines are based only on theory and expert opinion, as no clinical studies are available on this matter. Recommendations for attempting to prevent renal dysfunction associated with heart disease are mainly aimed at management of acute HF (see "Acute cardiovascular disorders causing acute kidney injury"). The recommendations for $CvRD_{CH}$ are (Vaden et al., 2017):

- Doses of diuretics, ACEIs, and positive inotropic agents should be tailored to each patient individually. Follow-up of dogs or cats should be performed 3 to 5 days after dose adjustments of these drugs, controlling kidney function, body weight, hydration status, electrolytes and systemic blood pressure.
- Spironolactone is a drug commonly used in chronic heart disease because of its benefits in preventing cardiac, renal, and vascular remodelling. Although it rarely occurs as a problem, the increase in plasma potassium concentration should be monitored when this drug is administered together with an ACEI, if renal dysfunction also exists.
- Systolic blood pressure should be maintained at normal levels, i.e. between 120 and 150 mmHg, to prevent hypotension and prevent or minimise target organ damage from hypertension.
- An important consequence to consider in $CvRD_{CH}$ patients is the alteration of the pharmacokinetics and pharmacodynamics of drugs due to cardiac or renal dysfunction; for instance, furosemide, which is actively secreted by the proximal tubule. Owing to the decrease in renal perfusion occurring during $CvRD_{CH}$, tubular damage occurs that reduces the expected response to diuretics. In addition, drugs that are excreted by the kidney, such as digoxin, enalapril, or atenolol, will require dose adjustment if a patient suffers from CKD in the context of $CvRD_{CH}$. In the case of patients receiving drugs highly bound to proteins such as pimobendan or digoxin for heart disease, their doses should be reviewed if there is also metabolic acidosis or hypoalbuminaemia due to CKD.
- Ensuring adequate nutritional intake is important for $CvRD_{CH}$ management. It would be advisable to offer these patients diets with moderate sodium restriction and to correct phosphorus and fatty acid ratios. Also, it should be noted that dogs in a very advanced stage of heart disease generally lose muscle mass and have a poor body condition, so one of the objectives to be achieved is adequate protein and energy intake. This is difficult as excessive protein and phosphorus intake contributes to the progression and worsening of kidney disease. It is therefore recommended to obtain the opinion of a nutrition expert.

04

CARDIOVASCULAR DISORDERS SECONDARY TO KIDNEY DISEASE

ACUTE KIDNEY DISEASE CONTRIBUTING TO IMPAIRED CARDIAC FUNCTION

M.ª Ángeles Daza González

CHRONIC KIDNEY DISEASE CONTRIBUTING TO IMPAIRED CARDIAC FUNCTION

Rafael Barrera Chacón • Javier Duque Carrasco

ACUTE KIDNEY DISEASE CONTRIBUTING TO IMPAIRED CARDIAC FUNCTION

Introduction

Accumulation of uraemic toxins, metabolic acidosis, electrolyte imbalances, and fluid overload are consequences of acute kidney injury (AKI). The high mortality associated with this injury cannot be explained only by a loss of kidney function or its complications, since communication between the kidney and other organs such as the lung, heart, brain, liver, and bowel may trigger multiorgan dysfunction (Fig. 1).

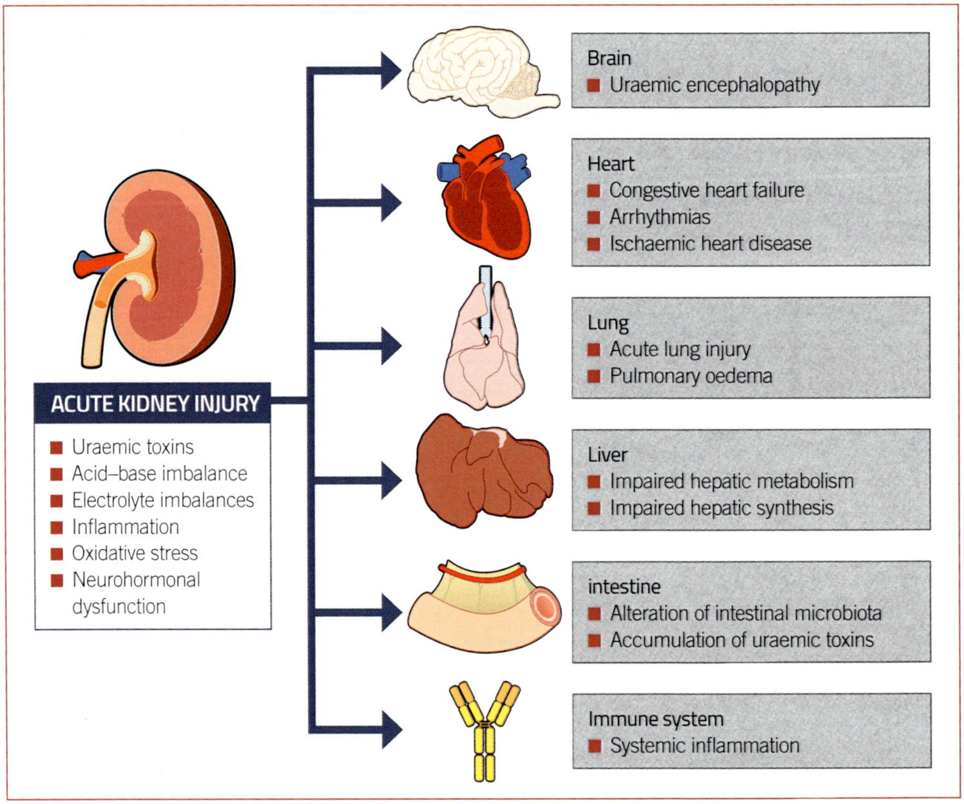

Figure 1. Impact of acute kidney injury (AKI) on distant organs.

Cardiovascular–renal disorders secondary to acute renal diseases ($CvRD_{AK}$) occur when AKI contributes to or precipitates the development of acute heart injury.

Acute kidney disease refers to AKI that can lead to poor functioning of the kidneys and subsequent inability to fulfil their excretory, metabolic and endocrine functions.

The International Renal Interest Society (IRIS) lists the AKI classification criteria on its website (http://www.iris-kidney.com/pdf/4_ldc-revised-grading-of-acute-kidney-injury.pdf).

As described in the chapter on $CvRD_{AH}$, acute heart failure is defined as the acute onset of clinical signs or rapid worsening of pre-existing heart failure requiring urgent treatment.

Aetiology

The most common causes of AKI are prerenal (e.g. inadequate intravascular volume due to translocation/loss of volume or vasodilation), renal (e.g. toxic), and postrenal (e.g. traumatic).

Pathophysiology

AKI causes cardiac dysfunction directly or indirectly through inflammatory mechanisms, oxidative stress, and neuroendocrine secretion (Fig. 2); as a result of fluid overload, electrolyte imbalances, and metabolic acidosis; and, finally, due to alteration of the pharmacokinetics of certain drugs (e.g. digoxin).

Direct effects of AKI on the heart

Immune system impairment

AKI can impair the cellular immune response, for example, by adhesion and extravasation of leukocytes in the kidney and in distal organs such as the heart. Neutrophils attached to the vascular endothelium release substances such as proteases and free radicals that induce direct tissue damage or stimulate the expression of cytokines that play a key role in heart failure.

Inflammation and oxidative stress

Cytokines released during experimental renal ischaemia have a direct cardiodepressant effect, including reduction of left ventricular ejection fraction. Nitrous oxide and free radicals also exert a negative inotropic effect. Inflammation associated with AKI can alter pulmonary vessel permeability, triggering interstitial oedema and bleeding.

Apoptosis

Apoptosis of myocardial cells and neutrophil activation contribute to tissue injury and lethal cardiac dysfunction after AKI.

Neurohormonal activation

Activation of the sympathetic nervous system (SNS) initially maintains cardiac output, but exerts harmful effects on the myocardium through different mechanisms, such as activation of the renin–angiotensin–aldosterone system (RAAS) and release of angiotensin II.

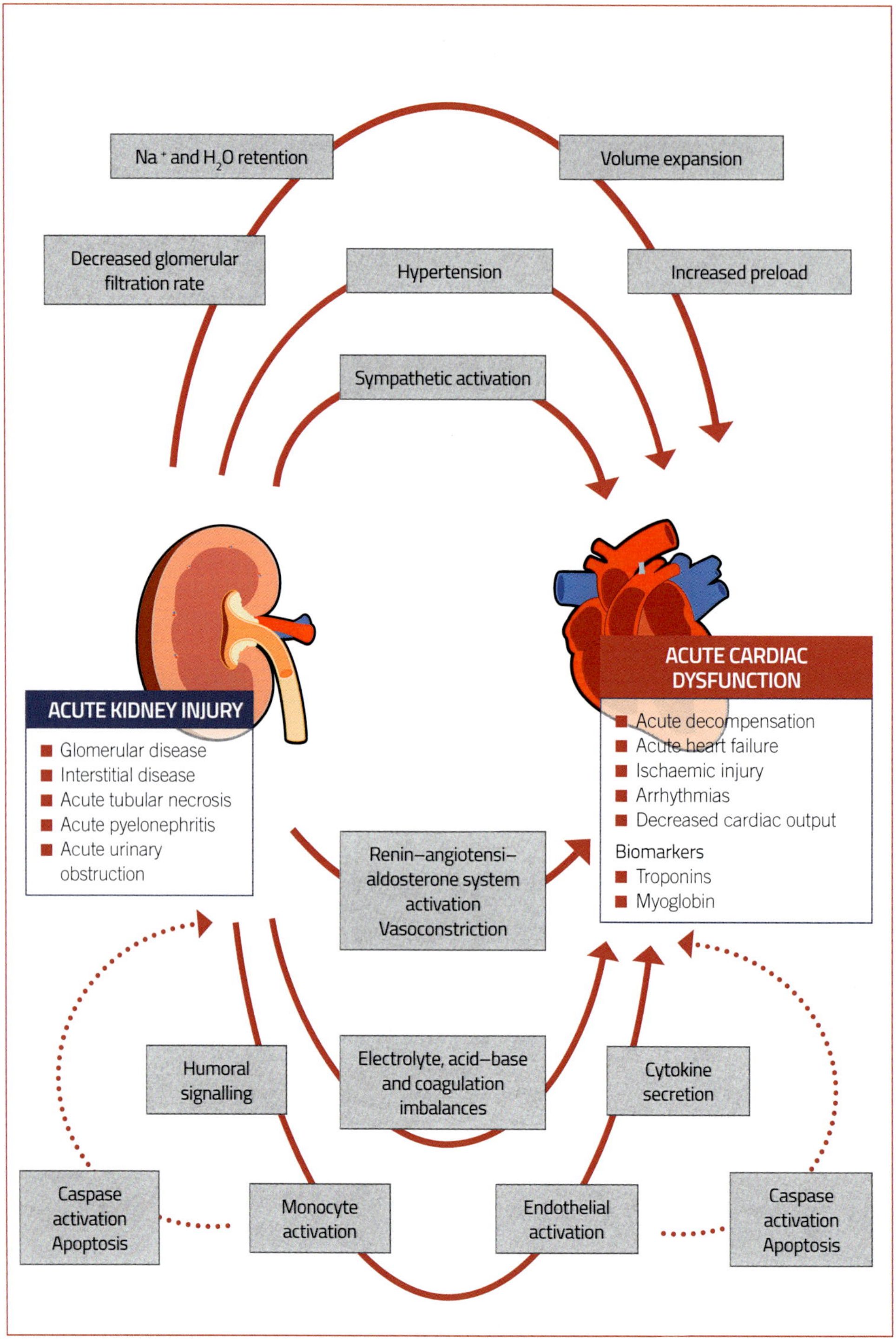

Figure 2. Pathophysiology of cardiovascular–renal type 3 syndrome or acute renocardiac syndrome.

Indirect effects of AKI on the heart

Fluid overload

Oliguria may lead to sodium and water retention, resulting in volume overload, hypertension, pulmonary oedema due to increased hydrostatic pressure, and myocardial dysfunction (Fig. 3).

Fluid overload is related to less favourable prognosis in critically ill patients, because renal function worsens from venous congestion.

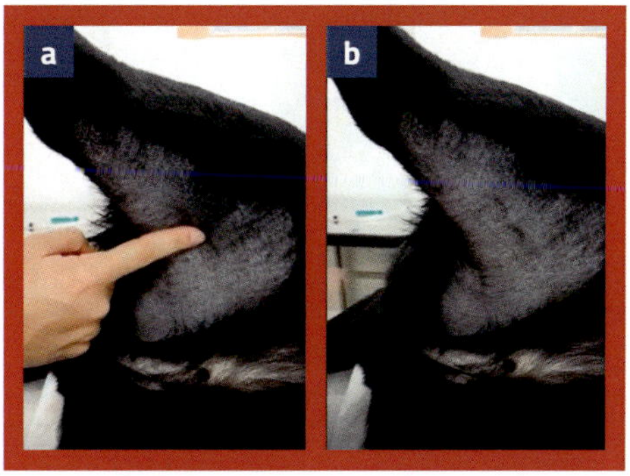

Figure 3. Digital pressure on the inside of the hind limb of a dog patient (a). Fovea due to fluid accumulation in tissues (b).

Electrolyte imbalances

Hyperkalaemia decreases resting membrane potential by increasing cell membrane excitability (Fig. 4). Electrocardiography (ECG) may reveal first-degree atrioventricular block, decreased or absent P wave amplitude, and ST segment depression. In the event of severe hyperkalaemia, some common ECG findings include bundle branch block, tachycardia and ventricular fibrillation, and idioventricular rhythms (Fig. 5).

Hypokalaemia (e.g. secondary to hyperaldosteronism) results in a more negative action potential and thereby reduces cell membrane excitability. Abnormalities in cardiac conduction, including increased QRS duration, increased P-wave duration and amplitude, prolonged PR interval, and atrioventricular block, can be observed on ECG (Fig. 6).

Calcium plays an important role in regulating the cardiac cycle. Hypercalcaemia may cause AKI and may manifest as bradycardia (with progression to asystole and cardiac arrest), PR interval prolongation, QRS complex widening, QT interval shortening, and ST-segment shortening or absence (Fig. 7).

Ethylene glycol poisoning may lead to AKI and hypocalcaemia because the antifreeze

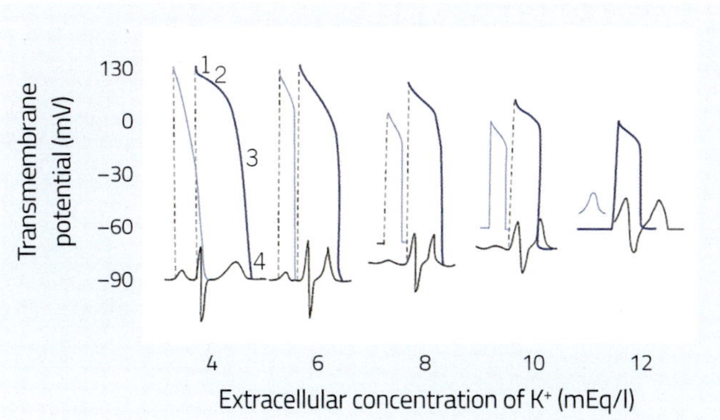

Figure 4. Diagram of the atrioventricular action potential superimposed on the ECG at different extracellular potassium concentrations (4, 6, 8, 10, and 12 mEq/l). The numbers on the left represent the transmembrane potential in millivolts (modified from El-Sherif and Turitto, 2011).

metabolites chelate calcium. In severely affected animals, it is possible to observe changes in inotropism or chronotropism and electrocardiographic signs such as ST segment and QT interval prolongation, and wide peaked T waves.

Hyperphosphataemia may cause arrhythmias, depress myocardial contractility and cause respiratory muscle weakness.

Acidosis

Acidosis may worsen pulmonary vasoconstriction, increase right ventricular afterload, and decrease myocardial contractility. In addition, acidosis increases the proportion of unbound calcium, worsening those clinical signs related with hypercalcaemia.

Uraemic toxins

Acute accumulation of uraemic toxins may directly affect myocardial cell contractility and lead to pericarditis, pericardial effusion, myocardial ischaemia, and organ dysfunction (Fig. 8).

Uraemia, systemic inflammation, and oxidative stress contribute to fluid accumulation within the lung, resulting in oedema that is not due to increased hydrostatic pressure and is also called "nephrogenic pulmonary oedema".

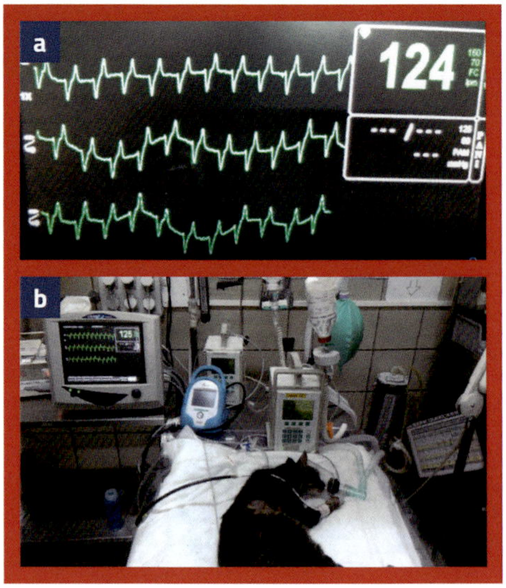

Figure 5. ECG in a patient with hyperkalaemia (K^+ >10 mEq/l) in which a right bundle branch block is observed (a). Treatment with sodium bicarbonate (b).

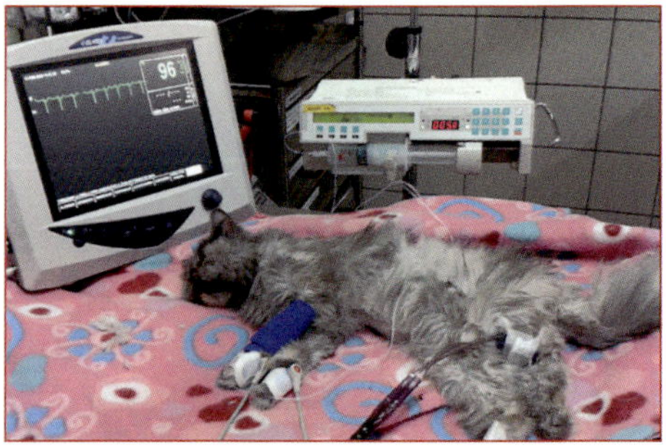

Figure 6. ECG of a cat with hypokalaemia (K^+=1.7 mEq/l) and treatment with potassium chloride.

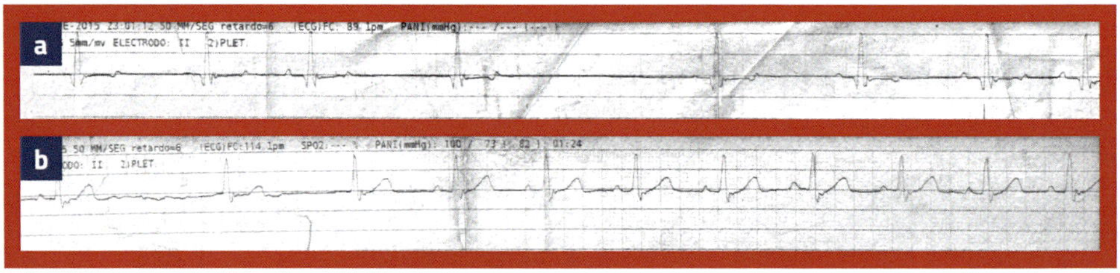

Figure 7. Pretreatment ECG of patient with hypercalcaemia (Ca^{2+} >2.5 mmol/l). A marked reduction in heart rate and an increase in ST segment duration (a) are seen. ECG of same patient after treatment with furosemide and corticosteroids (Ca^{2+}=1.38 mmol/l). Heart rate elevation and ST segment normalisation are seen (b).

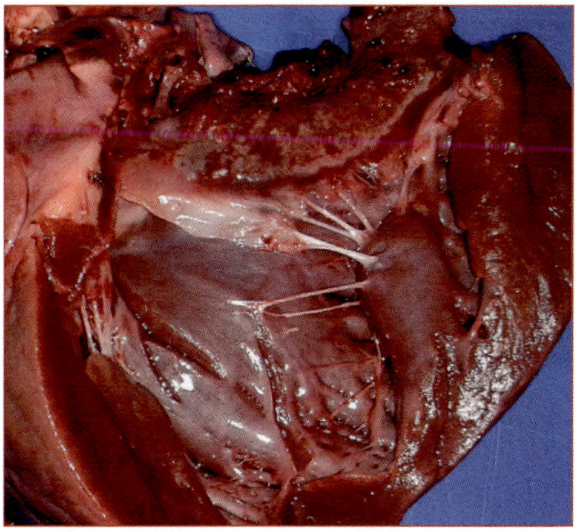

Figure 8. Uraemic endocarditis in a patient with acute kidney injury.

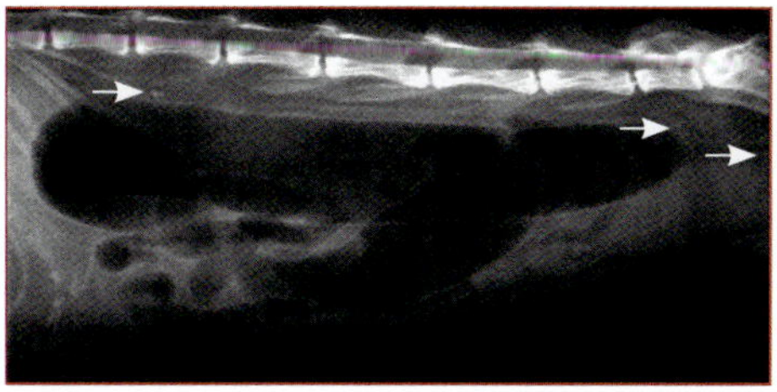

Figure 9. Lateral X-ray of the abdomen of a cat. The arrows show ureterolites in different segments of the ureter.

Diagnosis

Diagnostic imaging

Radiology

X-rays are useful to determine whether both kidneys are present and detect any changes in their size, silhouette, position, and radiographic density of the kidneys, as well as the presence of stones (Fig. 9).

To determine the size of the kidney, the length of the renal silhouette is compared with the vertebral body of the L2 vertebra. In healthy animals, the maximum length should be between 2.5–3.5 times the length of L2 in dogs and 2.4–3.0 times in cats. If both renal silhouettes are enlarged, the differential diagnosis includes neoplasm, polycystic kidney disease, and bilateral hydronephrosis. If one silhouette is enlarged and the other reduced, it is usually due to compensatory hypertrophy of the unaffected kidney.

As for the renal contour, the most common causes of change are polycystic disease, neoplasm, abscess, simple cyst, haematoma, or degenerative disease.

Ultrasound

Unlike X-rays, renal ultrasound offers information on its internal architecture.

Ultrasound examination of the kidney may help differentiate between an acute or chronic injury. For example, in chronic cases reduced-size kidneys of irregular contour, cortical hyperechogenicity, cystic lesions in the cortex with anechoic content, stones, etc., can be seen.

The presence of pyelectasia may be indicative of obstructive nephropathy (Fig. 10) or pyelonephritis (asymmetric dilatation), but it may also be due to fluid administration or use of diuretics (symmetrical dilation), etc.

The diagnosis of pyelonephritis cannot be made solely on the basis of the ultrasound findings; however, these findings are more robust if the patient shows compatible clinical signs such as polydipsia/polyuria or active urinary sediment.

The presence of a small amount of perirenal fluid should correlate with the appearance of the kidneys. This lesion may be indicative of leptospirosis, inflammation, intoxication and even lymphosarcoma.

Thoracic ultrasound can detect the presence of pulmonary oedema, pleural effusion, and pericardial effusion, among other signs.

Laboratory diagnosis

Cardiac biomarkers such as N-terminal pro–B-type natriuretic peptide (NT-proBNP) and cardiac troponin I (cTnI) may be determined to evaluate damage to the heart caused by renal disease.

Some difficulty exists in characterising some patients only based on the results of these tests due to the existence of grey zones. In addition, clinically relevant changes related to breed have been reported between healthy individuals, ill individuals, and between healthy and ill individuals.

On the other hand, it has been reported that plasma levels of these biomarkers are elevated in patients with acute or chronic kidney disease and apparently normal cardiac function. It is therefore difficult to establish whether elevation of the biomarker reflects the presence of cardiac damage or is a result of reduction of its excretion.

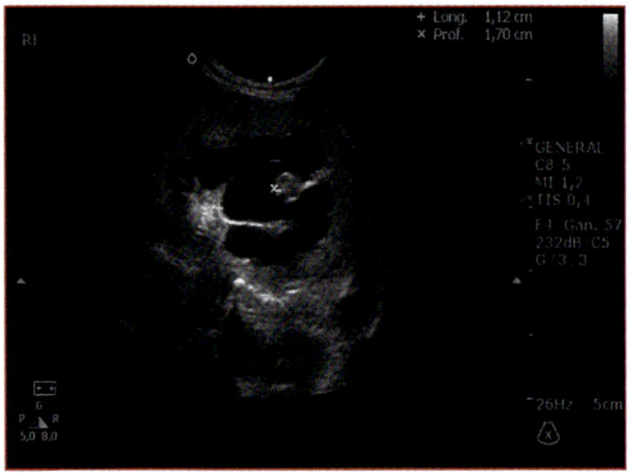

Figure 10. Renal ultrasound of a cat with pyelectasis and ureteral obstruction by a nephrolith.

Clinical management

The best treatment requires identifying patients in different disease states, for example, those at risk of developing AKI versus those who already have AKI and require renal replacement therapy (RRT).

By stage

High risk of acute kidney injury

Elderly, chronic kidney disease, heart failure, hypovolaemic, septic patients, etc. are considered at high risk of AKI.

At this stage it is important to avoid or minimise the use of nephrotoxic drugs and diuretics, as well as certain procedures (e.g. administration of X-ray contrast agents). Prevention of hypotension is vital for preventing AKI. It is therefore important to correct volume reduction together with administration of vasopressors to maintain mean arterial pressure.

Stage 1

Stage 1 includes patients with AKI who may develop renal failure. They should be treated in the same way as the previous group. It is also important to investigate and correct the predisposing causes, perform continuous monitoring and administer supportive therapy.

Stage 2 (injury)

Stage 2 patients are at high risk of morbidity and mortality, require conservative therapy and monitoring to achieve stabilisation. An optimum intravascular volume, mean arterial pressure (MAP), cardiac output and oxygen transport capacity should be achieved, ensuring electrolyte maintenance and acid–base balance, and administering the adequate dose of drugs ensuring they are within the therapeutic range.

Stage 3 (renal failure)

At this stage, the patient is at high risk of death and extrarenal complications. RRT should be considered if medical treatment does not work, if kidney injury is severe, or if there is a high risk of complications.

In this last stage, prevention of left ventricular volume overload is critical to maintain cardiac output and systemic perfusion.

Conservative treatment

For control of crises, different therapeutic approaches will be established to restore vascular volume and correct electrolyte imbalances and potential complications in other systems.

Fluid therapy

Fluid therapy is the most important treatment in AKI in order to improve renal perfusion, start diuresis, accelerate elimination of nephrotoxic substances and prevent renal tubular obstruction. Initial stabilisation with aggressive fluid therapy, followed by more restrictive maintenance, may decrease the incidence of AKI.

As regards the type of fluid to be used, balanced isotonic crystalloids are usually preferred, because they are alkalinising and thus improve acidosis and facilitate potassium translocation into the cell. For hypercalcaemia, 0.9 % sodium chloride is preferred. However, solutions with high chlorine content may cause kidney damage and worsen acidosis.

In case of haemorrhagic shock, administration of whole blood or packed red blood cells may be combined with crystalloids.

Starches are only considered when there is no response to crystalloids in nonseptic patients without renal failure.

Before any fluid is administered, it is important to collect a blood and urine sample to obtain baseline laboratory values.

Hypovolaemic shock

Targeted patient stabilisation will be performed by administering crystalloid boluses of 10–15 ml/kg in dogs and 5–10 ml/kg in cats. The efficacy of fluid replacement is assessed by evaluating the improvement of perfusion parameters, with the initial haemodynamic target being a mean arterial pressure (MAP) ≥65 mmHg, urine output >0.5 ml/kg/h, and normalisation of blood lactate. If a central catheter is available, central venous pressure (CVP) (Fig. 11), oxygen saturation in the vena cava ($S_{VC}O_2$) or mixed venous saturation (S_VO_2) can be measured. Monitor for signs of overload when doses of 90 ml/kg (dogs) or 60 ml/kg (cats) of crystalloids have been reached.

It is recommended to use vasopressor therapy (norepinephrine, vasopressin, or its synthetic analogue terlipressin, individually or in combination) rather than administering extra fluid volumes.

If a vasopressor is ineffective, adrenal insufficiency should be assessed. As a clinical test, hydrocortisone may be given at a dose of 0.5–1 mg/kg every 6 hours IV, and methylprednisolone or prednisolone sodium succinate may be given at an initial dose of 1 mg/kg IV, followed by 0.25 mg/kg every 6 hours.

Absence of hypovolaemic shock

In this case, fluid therapy will be governed by the following approach:

- The **deficit volume** will be determined by the following equation:

% dehydration × weight (kg) × 1000 = deficit in ml

This deficit will be replaced with a balanced electrolyte solution over 2–8 hours to restore renal perfusion. If no dehydration is detected, subclinical dehydration of 3–5 % will be assumed. In animals with cardiovascular compromise, the deficit must be replaced in 8–12 hours or 12–24 hours and low-sodium fluids must be used. If oliguria is corrected after administration of the deficit, the maintenance volume will be administered together with the volume of pathological losses.

- **Daily maintenance volume.** Once the patient is hydrated, the volume corresponding to physiological fluid losses will be administered:

Patients weighing <2 kg:
$70 \times \text{weight (kg)}^{0.75} = \text{ml/day}$

Patients weighing between 2 and 70 kg:
$30 \times \text{weight (kg)} + 70 = \text{ml/day}$

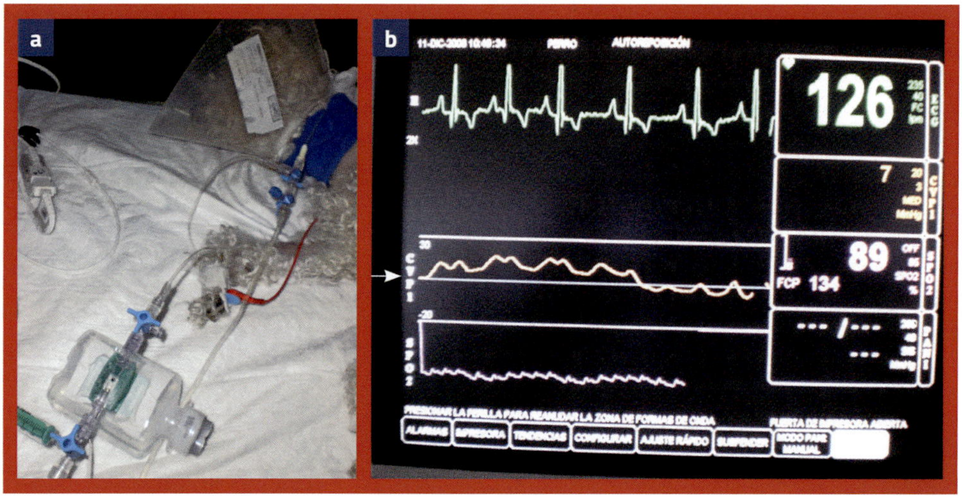

Figure 11. Central venous catheter and blood pressure transducer in a patient with acute renocardiac syndrome (a). Graph of central venous pressure (CVP) (white arrow) (b).

In this stage, it is important to use crystalloids with low sodium concentrations (40–60 mEq/l). Fluid administration should not be continued in an attempt to establish urine flow when the requirements have already been administered. Fluid therapy should be discontinued if signs of fluid overload or 10 % weight gain are observed, unless this is the calculation of the deficit.

- **Volume of pathological losses.** Losses due to vomiting and diarrhoea should be replaced with an isotonic crystalloid solution. For this, fluid intakes (e.g. fluid therapy, medications, etc.), fluid losses (e.g. diuresis), and patient weight should be assessed daily to avoid overhydration.

Fluid therapy should be discontinued over 2–3 days, once the level of uraemic toxins is not reduced within 24 hours.

Hyperkalaemia

It should be treated whenever ECG signs are observed:

- Treat the triggering problem; for example, restore diuresis in oliguria/anuria and recannulate the urethra in case of obstruction (Fig. 12).
- Remove any sources of potassium or drugs that contribute to the development of hyperkalaemia (e.g. ACEIs).
- 10 % calcium gluconate or calcium chloride: does not affect K^+ plasma levels, but blocks its cardiotoxic effects. The dose of calcium gluconate is 0.5–1.5 ml/kg and the dose of calcium chloride is 0.2 ml/kg infused over 5–10 minutes with ECG monitoring.
- Glucose: promotes the release of endogenous insulin causing movement of K^+ into the cell. Doses of 0.7–1 g/kg of 50 % glucose are usually given over 3–5 minutes.

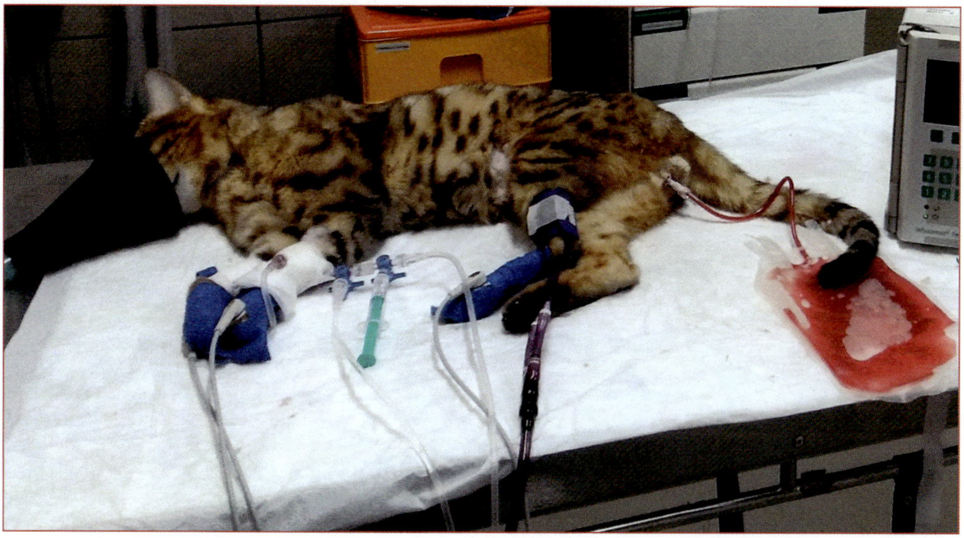

Figure 12. Urethral catheterisation in a cat with obstructive lower urinary tract disease (FLUTD).

- Insulin + glucose: 0.5 IU/kg regular insulin plus 2 g 50 % glucose (4 ml 50 % glucose) per insulin unit.
- Sodium bicarbonate: causes entry of K^+ into the cell when exchanged for H^+. It is usually administered at a dose of 1–2 mEq/kg over 20–30 minutes and may be redosed if necessary.
- Loop diuretics and thiazide diuretics increase tubular flow and potassium secretion.
- Salbutamol: 4 µg/kg IV over 20 minutes diluted in 5–10 ml dextrose in water or 2.5–5 mg nebulised over 10 minutes.
- Cation exchange resins (calcium polystyrene sulfonate): each gram binds 1 mEq of K^+ and releases 1–3 mEq of Na^+ in the gastrointestinal tract.
- If necessary, apply RRT.

Hypokalaemia

When replenishing potassium levels, it should be taken into account not to exceed doses of 0.5 mEq/kg/h, although in severe hypokalaemia 1–1.5 mEq/kg/h may be administered under ECG control (Fig. 13).

Acidosis

Acidosis should be treated if peripheral arterial pressure is <7.2 or bicarbonate concentration is <12 mEq/l.

Bicarbonate dose (mmol) =
3 × weight (kg) × base deficit

From 50 % to 60 % of the calculated dose will be administered over 30 minutes in order to prevent the development of metabolic alkalosis. The pH and bicarbonate will be analysed

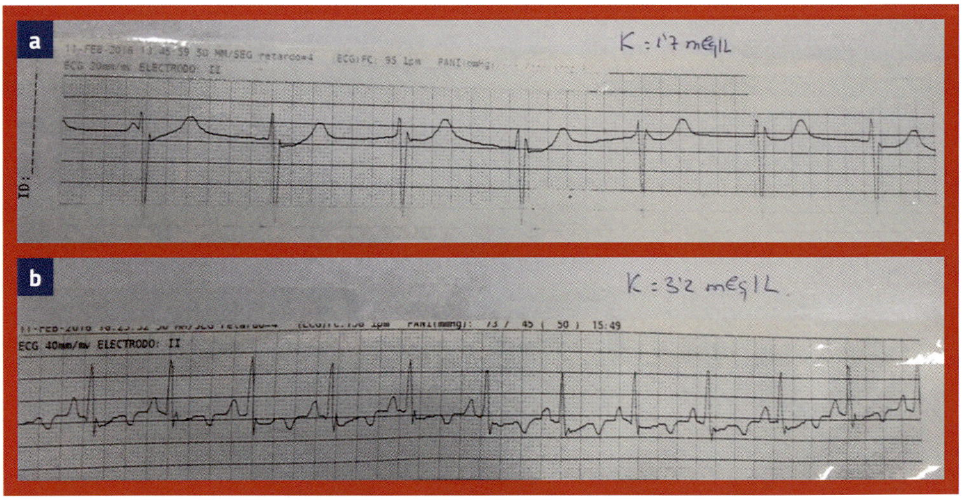

Figure 13. ECG of cat in Figure 6 before (a) and after (b) treatment with potassium chloride. Before treatment, bradycardia, a possible atrioventricular block (a P wave with a shortened PR interval is seen in the first complex and in all other complexes the P wave is not identified and may be included in the T wave or in the QRS complexes), and intrafascicular block (HR: 95 bpm) are seen. After treatment, normal sinus rhythm and possible QT interval prolongation are observed.

at 60 minutes and if the initial status persists, the remaining 50 % will be administered over 12–24 hours. Administration of sodium bicarbonate reduces the fraction of ionised calcium.

Hypercalcaemia

Management of hypercalcaemia includes:

- Fluid therapy: the goal is to correct dehydration, as haemoconcentration contributes to increased calcium levels.
- Diuretics: once rehydration is completed, administration of loop diuretics such as furosemide can promote calciuresis, subsequently replacing fluid loss according to "intakes and losses". An initial dose will be administered as a bolus dose of 1–2 mg/kg IV followed by an infusion of 1 mg/kg/h.
- Glucocorticoids: decrease serum calcium levels by preventing both calcium reabsorption in bone and intestine and increasing renal excretion. Dexamethasone: 0.10–0.22 mg/kg every 12 hours SC or IV; prednisone: 1.0–2.2 mg/kg every 12 hours PO, SC, or IV.
- Calcitonin: decreases serum calcium levels by decreasing osteoclast activity. The recommended dose is 4–6 IU/kg SC every 6–8 hours.
- Bisphosphonates: reduce serum calcium levels by decreasing osteoclastic activity one to two days after administration.

Hypocalcaemia

It can be controlled with calcium gluconate (0.5–1.5 ml/kg IV) administered over 10–20 minutes and under ECG control or with calcium chloride.

Hyperphosphataemia

Restoration of glomerular filtration rate increases phosphorus excretion. Oral phosphorus binders are only feasible in patients without uraemic syndrome. In case of oliguria/anuria, RRT should be used.

Recovery of diuresis

If oliguria persists after rehydration is completed, a small expansion of plasma volume may be considered by administering fluids at a rate of 3 % of the animal's weight. Diuretics may also be considered, taking into account that while improving urine output, diuretics do not improve renal function:

- Furosemide: initial loading bolus of 2–4 mg/kg IV in dogs and 2 mg/kg in cats. If there is a response at 30–60 minutes, consider continuous infusion of 0.25–1.0 mg/kg/h.
- Mannitol: not recommended in human patients for the treatment of acute anuria secondary to tubular necrosis due to renal ischaemia. It is administered in doses of 0.25–0.5 g/kg IV over 15-20 minutes. If there is a response, it should be repeated every 4–6 hours or given as a continuous infusion at a dose of 1–2 mg/kg/min without exceeding 2 g/kg/24 hours. It should not be administered in patients who are overhydrated, dehydrated, hyperosmolar, bleeding, with immunomediated haemolytic anaemia, pulmonary or interstitial oedema, vasculitis or heart failure.

Management of respiratory problems

Respiratory signs can be relieved by administering diuretics to treat fluid overload or lung oedema and pleural/pericardial effusion drainage.

Management of hypertension

It consists of avoiding volume overload or treating it if already present. Among the most commonly used agents are calcium channel blockers (amlodipine) and hydralazine.

Management of gastrointestinal signs

The gastric protectors considered most effective are proton pump inhibitors such as omeprazole. The most commonly used antiemetics are maropitant and metoclopramide.

Renal replacement therapy

RRT is indicated when anuria/oliguria, volume overload or hyperkalemia cannot be effectively controlled with medical therapy alone (Figs. 14 and 15). Delay in the start of RRT causes a worsening of renal failure that may be potentially irreversible.

When proposing such therapies, rather than considering any numerical value, disease progression, clinical status, and prognosis should be considered.

Such treatments are reserved for patients in whom there is the possibility of reversing the underlying kidney disease or improving the uraemic state.

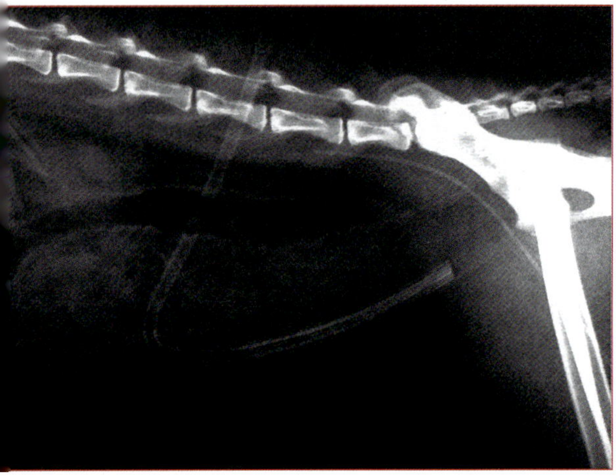

Figure 14. Central venous catheter and peritoneal drainage in a cat with acute kidney injury from lily poisoning.

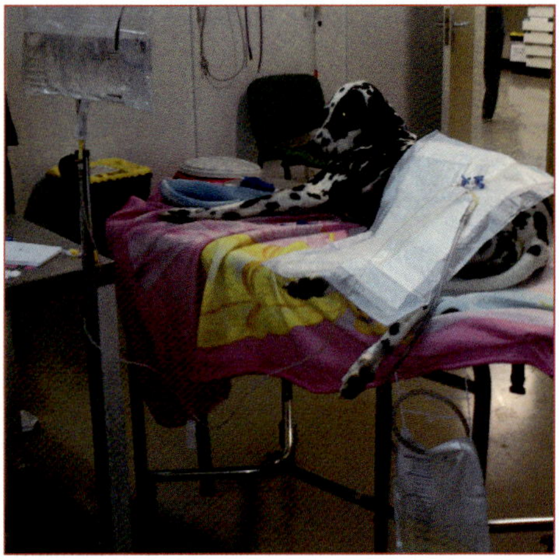

Figure 15. Peritoneal dialysis in a dog with grape poisoning.

CHRONIC KIDNEY DISEASE CONTRIBUTING TO IMPAIRED CARDIAC FUNCTION

Introduction

The most common kidney conditions in humans are glomerular disease, diabetic nephropathy, hypertensive nephropathy, nephrosclerosis, interstitial nephritis, and polycystic kidneys. However, the most common conditions reported in dogs are glomerular disease, pyelonephritis (Fig. 1) and acute tubular necrosis, while in cats, the most common condition is idiopathic chronic kidney disease (CKD), often characterised by tubulointerstitial fibrosis of unknown origin (Vaden et al., 2017). However, there is serious evidence to suggest that some of the mechanisms described in human CKD may occur in dogs and cats, and the clinical experience of veterinary hospitals supports this.

CKD is the most commonly diagnosed condition affecting the kidneys of dogs and cats. These animals experience progressive loss of functional nephrons, and the observed clinical manifestations tend to reflect the extent of renal injury even better than the study of structural lesions.

In most cases, it is usually irreversible and progressive, even with treatment. Prerenal, renal, and postrenal components sometimes develop that complicate the condition with an added acute condition, which may be reversible. However, even if these potential complications are corrected, they do not usually result in an improvement in renal function because

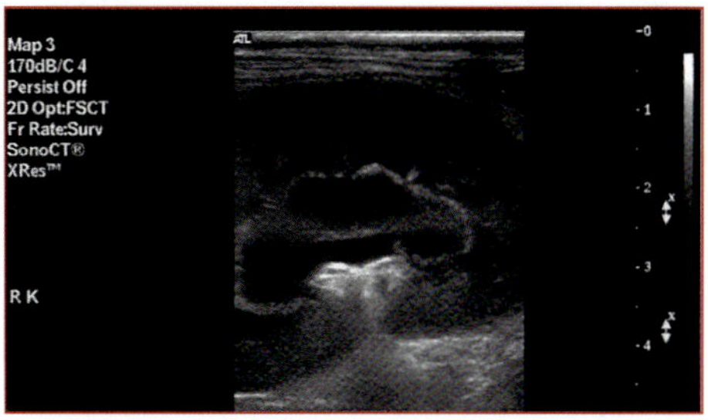

Figure 1. Ultrasound image corresponding to the right kidney of a 5-year-old Beagle dog with chronic kidney disease secondary to pyelonephritis.

the same compensatory and adaptive mechanisms designed to maintain renal function promote progressive loss of the remaining nephrons and impaired renal function.

The most widely accepted classification from the practical viewpoint is that developed by the International Renal Interest Society (IRIS; http://www.iris-kidney.com/guidelines/index.html), to aid clinicians in selecting treatment and appropriate patient follow-up (Table 1). In addition, it is completed with two subclassifications based on protein:creatinine ratio (UP:C) and systemic blood pressure (Table 2 and Table 3). This classification is very useful in the study of possible cases of cardiovascular–renal disorder.

In most cases, the disease is diagnosed when the first clinical signs occur (weight loss, apathy, and polyuria/polydipsia), which coincides with an increase in blood creatinine levels above the normal range.

Table 1. Adaptation of the classification established by the International Renal Interest Society (IRIS) for CKD in dogs and cats based on blood creatinine concentration.

Stage	Blood creatinine (µmol/l; mg/dl)		Comments
	Dogs	Cats	
At risk	<125; <1.4	<140; <1.6	Animals at risk of developing CKD due to different factors, e.g. exposure to nephrotoxic drugs, breed, living in geographic areas with a high prevalence of infectious diseases, and advanced age.
1	<125; <1.4	<140; <1.6	Nonazotaemic. With any renal abnormality present, e.g. inadequate urinary concentration with no identifiable nonrenal cause, abnormal renal palpation, abnormal renal findings on diagnostic imaging, proteinuria of renal origin, abnormal renal biopsy results, increased blood creatinine concentration in multiple serial samples.
2	125–180; 1.4–2.0	140–250; 1.6–2.8	Mild renal azotaemia: the lower limit of the range is within the reference values of many laboratories. Clinical signs often mild or absent.
3	181–440; 2.1–5.0	251–440; 2.9–5.0	Moderate renal azotaemia. Extrarenal clinical signs sometimes present, but their severity may vary. If there are no clinical signs, the case can be considered as early IRIS stage 3, whereas the presence of systemic signs can be considered as late IRIS stage 3.
4	>440; >5	>440; >5	Increasing risk of systemic clinical signs and uraemic crises.

Table 2. Adaptation of the classification established by the International Renal Interest Society (IRIS) for CKD according to proteinuria (UP:C value).

UP:C		Subclassification
Dogs	Cats	
<0.2	<0.2	Nonproteinuric
0.2–0.5	0.2–0.4	Borderline proteinuric
>0.5	>0.4	Proteinuric

Table 3. Adaptation of the classification established by the International Renal Interest Society (IRIS) for CKD based on blood pressure values.

Systolic blood pressure (mm Hg)	Blood pressure substaging	Risk of producing target organ damage
<140	Normotensive	Minimal
140–159	Prehypertensive	Low
160–179	Hypertensive	Moderate
>180	Severe hypertensive	High

When this occurs, glomerular filtration rate (GFR) has decreased to less than 75 % of its normal values, and at least three quarters of the nephrons are no longer functional. As a result, diagnosis of CKD is usually made late. Consideration should also be given to the hyperbolic behaviour of creatinine in relation to GFR (Fig. 2). When the latter is not yet very affected, slight increases in creatinine concentration may indicate a serious worsening in renal function.

Aetiology

It is difficult to assign specific aetiological causes to CKD, because the responsible cause is often undiagnosed or has even disappeared. Predisposing conditions such as advanced age, prior renal damage (congenital), and genetic factors may be present. Triggering factors such as immune-mediated diseases, parasitic diseases (leishmaniasis), systemic infections, urinary tract infections, urinary lithiasis, nephrotoxic drugs, hypertensive diseases, chronic hypoperfusion, neoplasms and amyloidosis must then occur (Polzin, 2011). From this point on, the disease progresses due to intrinsic mechanisms that develop and self-perpetuate the disease, causing progressive nephron destruction. The consequence is the development of chronic tubulointerstitial nephritis, glomerulonephritis and, less commonly, amyloidosis, in both dogs and cats.

Rather than aetiological causes, the pathophysiological mechanisms derived from CKD, and especially those that may involve the cardiovascular system, should be considered. The most common mechanisms are hypertension and uraemia, and in advanced stages, electrolyte imbalances and plasma volume abnormalities. In addition, in patients with previous cardiac disease under treatment, poisoning by certain drugs (digoxin, enalapril, and atenolol) should be considered.

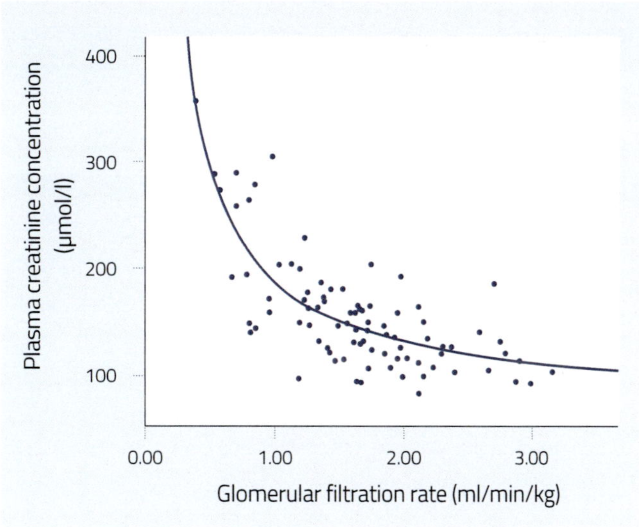

Figure 2. Relationship between plasma creatinine concentration (µmol/l) and glomerular filtration rate (ml/min/kg) in cats (taken from Finch, 2014).

Pathophysiology

$CvRD_{CK}$ refers to a cardiovascular injury or dysfunction caused by a primary kidney disease, and is less common than $CvRD_{CH}$ (Ronco et al., 2008). In human medicine, it is accepted that CKD involves the convergence between traditional and nontraditional cardiovascular risk factors (anaemia, uraemia, hyperphosphataemia, secondary hyperparathyroidism, coronary and valve calcifications, hyperhomocysteinaemia, inflammation, and increased oxidative stress) (Cheung et al., 2004; Fonarow et al., 2005; El Nahas, 2010). The pathophysiological mechanisms involving the cardiovascular system whose origin may be the kidney in dogs and cats are not completely clear, but it is postulated that they may be those described below.

Systemic hypertension

From 30 % to 50 % of dogs with CKD have hypertension, mainly attributed to glomerular disease. According to IRIS, antihypertensive treatment is indicated in patients with a systemic blood pressure >160 mmHg (hypertensive or severely hypertensive animals; Table 3), because they are at greater risk of damage to target organs (Coleman and Brown, 2017), including the heart. Clinical manifestations include progressive kidney injury, acute blindness, hyphaema, retinal haemorrhage, retinal detachment, left ventricular hypertrophy, myocardial ischaemia, hypertensive encephalopathy (intermittent confusion, depression and collapse), dementia and cerebrovascular haemorrhage, responsible for seizures, coma, and death (Brown, 2011; Stepien, 2011).

The proposed pathophysiological mechanisms of systemic hypertension in animals with CKD include alterations in renal sodium regulation, activation of the renin–angiotensin–aldosterone system (RAAS), and excessive activity of the sympathetic nervous system. Due to increased sodium and water retention and arteriolar vasoconstriction, these mechanisms may contribute to the development of systemic hypertension by increasing blood volume, cardiac output and systemic vascular resistance (Syme, 2011).

Uraemia

Uraemia directly affects myocardial contractility through the accumulation of depressant factors, particularly when pericarditis is present (an uncommon condition in veterinary medicine). In human medicine it has been shown to induce cardiomyocyte loss, with diffuse interstitial fibrosis and hypertrophy of the remaining myocytes, as well as microvascular disease (Sultán and Osso, 2006) and a progressive decrease in contractile capacity.

Electrolyte abnormalities

As glomerular filtration rate decreases, functional nephrons become overloaded and unable to maintain water and electrolyte excretion. However, the body's electrolyte balance is preserved by decreasing tubular reabsorption. This balance is maintained until GFR is less than 80 %. Although compensatory mechanisms in the kidney are able to maintain the balance until advanced stages of the disease, a time is reached when they are insufficient and fail in the end stages of the disease. This is when hyperkalaemia can develop, often coinciding with oliguria/ oligoanuria, indicative of these stages. Hyperkalaemia can in turn be responsible for cardiac rhythm and conduction disorders; a life-threatening ventricular arrhythmia may even occur.

Hypokalaemia is uncommon in CKD. However, it may occur, mainly due to the decreased appetite associated with the disease, especially in cats, with an incidence of 20–30 % (DiBartola et al., 1987; Elliot and Barber 1998). It is actually probably due to a combination of appetite loss and increased renal losses as a result of polyuria. Its consequences on the cardiovascular system are uncommon, and when they occur, they consist of cardiac arrhythmias due to late ventricular repolarisation, particularly in patients with pre-existing heart disease.

Plasma volume abnormalities

Fluid balance is maintained for a long time in dogs and cats with CKD, provided drinking water is available and it is not complicated by acute prerenal disease due to dehydration. However, a patient's fluid volume and haemodynamic status may be altered in case of severe or advanced CKD. In these stages, urine production is decreased, which may lead to volume overload that contributes to the development of vascular congestion. Its detrimental effect on cardiac function is particularly evident in dogs and cats that are already suffering from valve disease, diastolic dysfunction or anaemia secondary to kidney disease.

Uraemic patients usually experience anorexia, hypodipsia, and vomiting, which may contribute to decreased plasma volume and decreased cardiac output. Additionally, in cases of uraemic gastroenteritis, an acute episode of vomiting may promote greater vagal stimulation, causing bradycardia and triggering in severe cases cardiac arrest (Brown, 2011; Stepien, 2011).

Drug toxicity

When kidney function is not adequate, special attention should be paid to the administration of renally excreted drugs, e.g. digoxin, particularly in patients with cardiac diseases. Approximately two thirds of the drug is renally excreted. Its clearance is proportional to that of creatinine, so in patients with decreased renal function its half-life increases and it is necessary to reduce the dose or switch to a drug with a different elimination route. The same occurs with other drugs such as enalapril, whose renal excretion reaches 94 % of the drug, and atenolol, with a renal excretion of 40 %–50 %. Primary renal dysfunction may lead to signs of toxicity from these drugs, including arrhythmias, hypotension and worsening of myocardial function.

Anaemia

Normocytic, normochromic, and nonregenerative anaemia is very common in dogs and cats with established CKD. It is caused by a deficiency in renal erythropoietin production, decreased erythrocyte half-life, nutritional abnormalities (iron, vitamin B_{12} and folate deficiency), renal erythropoietin inhibitory factors in uraemic plasma, blood loss, and myelofibrosis.

In human medicine, it is accepted that it may have a negative effect on cardiac function (cardiorenal anaemia). It produces a state of cardiac hypoxia that may be responsible for the death of cardiomyocytes, causing pathological remodelling of the heart and a process of oxidative stress, which contributes to cell damage and stimulates the RAAS. The combination of chronically reduced renal function and persistent anaemia can lead to left ventricular hypertrophy and systolic function deficit. However, in dogs and cats it does not appear to play a significant role in the development of secondary cardiovascular diseases, because it is usually mild or moderate, unless there are concurrent factors such as chronic inflammation, neoplasms, etc. (Carlos Sampedrano et al., 2006; Chetboul et al., 2003; Henik et al., 2004). In people, erythropoietin has been shown to prevent apoptosis and increase the number of myocytes (Tang et al., 2008).

Canine leishmaniasis

CKD is a serious complication of canine leishmaniosis, and concomitant heart damage (myocarditis) may be found, revealed by increased troponin levels in the blood. Mild myocardial damage may occur early and become severe in dogs with advanced disease. However, when CKD develops, it seems unlikely that a concurrent azotaemic state or development of systemic hypertension and anaemia are important factors in the development of myocardial damage (Martínez et al., 2016).

Diagnosis

When abnormalities of the cardiovascular system are detected, it is difficult to know if they are secondary to CKD ($CvRD_{CK}$), if CKD is secondary to cardiovascular disease ($CvRD_{CH}$), or if they are concomitant ($CvRD_{HK}$).

A complete physical examination, blood pressure measurement, imaging, and laboratory blood and urine tests should be performed in all animals. Electrocardiography is also indicated for electrolyte imbalances.

Blood pressure measurement

The IRIS provides useful indications for interpretation in dogs, and recommends several measurements on different days or at least two hours apart (Table 3).

Unlike in human medicine, where the most commonly diagnosed cause is primary (essential) hypertension, in canine and feline medicine CKD is the most common cause. However, there is no clear correlation between severity and degree of hypertension (Finco, 2004). Thus, hypertension may develop in subclinical renal diseases or even in early stages. This relationship is less clear in cats than in dogs. The presence of hypertension is associated with worsening proteinuria, which in turn aggravates CKD (Chakrabarti et al., 2012).

Although the studies published on its incidence in dogs and cats with CKD have yielded a wide variety of results, they all agree that it is high (Buranakarl et al., 2007; Kobayashi et al., 1990; Syme et al., 2002). Therefore, blood pressure should be measured in all affected dogs and cats, and particularly in those with suspected glomerular disease. However, it should not be forgotten that there are nonrenal causes responsible for hypertensive states, such as diabetes mellitus, hyperaldosteronism, hyperadrenocorticism, adrenal pheochromocytomas, fluid administration in patients with kidney disease and administration of some drugs (erythropoietin and erythropoietin stimulating agents, dopamine, glucocorticoids, and mineralocorticoids) (Segev, 2017).

Cardiac damage secondary to hypertension, usually manifested as ventricular hypertrophy, is presumably the least important of target organ damage (ocular lesions are more common). Clinical signs due to heart failure secondary to hypertension are rarely documented, because left ventricular hypertrophy is usually not severe enough to cause signs detected by the owner. However, hypertension can exacerbate the existing heart disease (Segev, 2017).

Finally, mention should be made of arterial hypotension (systolic pressure <90 mmHg), an uncommon condition in CKD. It may cause decreased cardiac output, tissue perfusion and GFR, and activate nonadaptive neurohormonal responses (Morales et al., 2002).

Electrocardiography

Electrocardiographic changes associated with hyperkalaemia in small animals begin when serum potassium levels exceed 6.5–7.0 mmol/l. They initially include increased T wave amplitude, shortening of the QT interval, and flattening of the P wave. Progression of hyperkalaemia leads to prolongation of the PR interval and widening of the QRS complex. Severe hyperkalaemia decreases P wave amplitude due to decreased conduction in the atria. If atrial conduction ceases, the P wave disappears and significant bradycardia develops. If this continues, the QRS complex gradually widens until it fuses with the T wave to form a sinusoidal wave, a sign of imminent cardiac arrest (DiBartola and de Morais, 2006).

Electrocardiographic changes associated with hypokalaemia are uncommon: QT prolongation, ST segment deviations, and decreased T wave amplitude.

Diagnostic imaging

Radiographic examination is useful for detecting changes in heart shape, vascular structures, and pulmonary parenchymal pattern. Echocardiography is used to assess cardiac morphology and function. The B-, M-, and Doppler modes (spectral, flow and tissue) allow specific information to be obtained about blood flow velocity and direction, movement of the different cardiac structures or wall thickness (Chetboul and Tissier, 2012), as well as a number of measures and indices to be determined that provide information about the possible existence of different cardiac diseases.

Radiographically, the kidneys are often normal in CKD. When changes occur, they are usually bilateral, but they may be asymmetrical. Small, irregular or deformed kidneys and images consistent with areas of mineralisation or stones may be seen. For more accurate measures and observations, excretory urography may be used.

Ultrasound allows visualisation of abnormalities in the renal parenchyma and renal pelvis (Figs. 3 and 4), kidney stones (Fig. 5), and measures renal artery resistance and pulsatility indices. Computed tomography and magnetic resonance imaging may be used for more advanced studies.

Laboratory tests

Laboratory data confirm CKD and provide information on severity, course and prognosis. Assessment of renal filtration capacity is initially performed based on blood urea (or blood urea nitrogen [BUN]) and creatinine levels and urine protein assessment (UP:C ratio, microalbuminuria test, or urinary immunoglobulin G level). The concentration capacity of the kidney should preferably be tested by measuring urinary osmolality. However, because of the equipment required for its determination, density measurement is usually used.

The information provided by the above biomarkers is usually late, and it is important to obtain information earlier in order to start appropriate treatment and prevent complications, including those affecting the cardiovascular system.

The IRIS reports that earlier biomarkers are needed and recommends measuring the blood concentration of symmetrical dimethylarginine (SDMA), but also specifies that further field information is needed.

Plasma cystatin C, an indicator of glomerular damage, is currently under study.

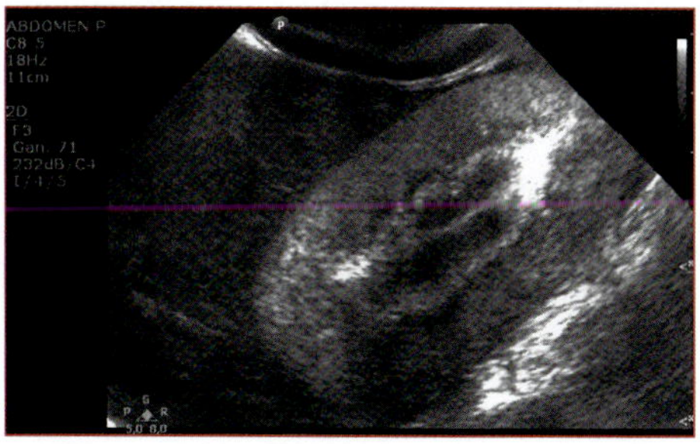

Figure 3. Ultrasound image of the left kidney of a 7-year-old French Bulldog female dog with chronic kidney disease showing hyperechogenicity of the renal cortex and mineralisation sites within it.

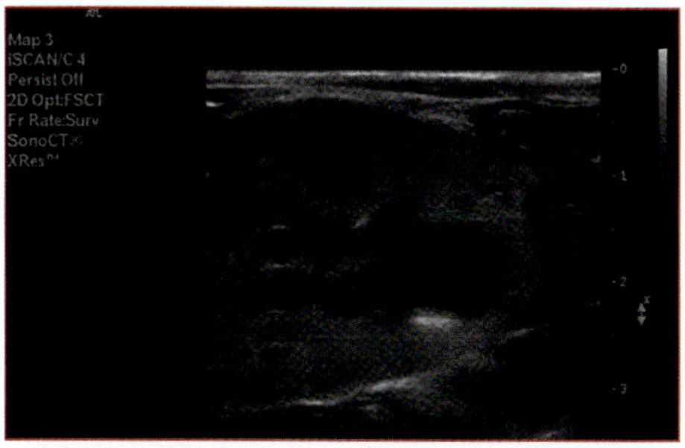

Figure 4. Ultrasound image of the left kidney of a 6-year-old Persian cat with chronic kidney disease secondary to polycystic kidney disease.

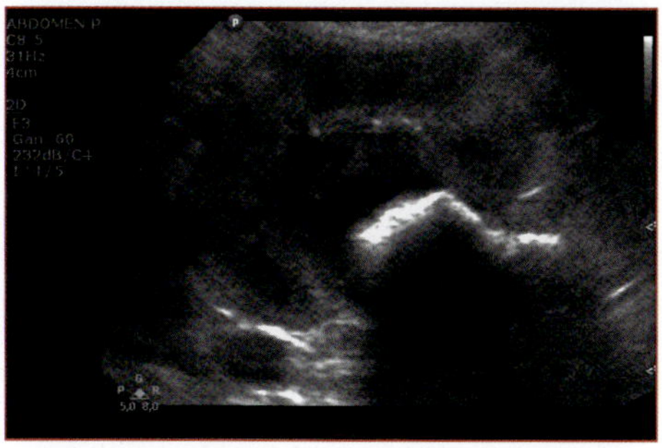

Figure 5. Ultrasound image of the left kidney of a 9-year-old Yorkshire Terrier male dog with chronic kidney disease secondary to kidney stones.

In human medicine, it is considered an earlier biomarker than creatinine. However, this could not be verified in canine medicine.

Measurement of tubular biomarkers, traditionally associated with acute kidney injury, is also important because glomerular processes eventually develop into mixed (glomerular and tubular) processes. These biomarkers may serve as earlier biomarkers than those traditionally used. Most are still in the study phase, but the results obtained appear to be promising. The following can be mentioned: fractional excretion of electrolytes, N-acetyl-β-D-glucosaminidase (NAG), urinary cystatin C, retinol binding protein (RBP), γ-glutamyl transpeptidase (GGT), neutrophil gelatinase-associated lipocalin (NGAL), and clusterin.

Cardiovascular impairment in dogs and cats with CKD is not easily demonstrated by laboratory tests. Blood concentrations of N-terminal pro–B-type natriuretic peptide (NT-proBNP), B-type natriuretic peptide (BNP), N-terminal pro-atrial natriuretic peptide (NT-proANP) and cardiac troponin I (cTnI), biomarkers studied in primary cardiovascular diseases, may be used. However, interpretation is sometimes difficult, particularly with regard to cardiovascular changes secondary to CKD. This is because these biomarkers show changes depending on the heart's condition at each time, they show individual and breed variations in both healthy and diseased animals, some of them are partly dependent on renal function for excretion, and there are few studies of cases associated with $CvRD_{CK}$ in these species (Pouchelon et al., 2015). It is therefore difficult to know if their increase reflects heart injury, normal variation or a decrease in their excretion. This is evident in cases of leishmaniasis, because the disease itself is able to increase the blood value of cardiac biomarkers, even when there is no evidence in CKD.

Therefore, it is easy to demonstrate the presence of CKD in dogs and cats using laboratory methods, but it is difficult to know whether kidney disease is primary, secondary to heart disease, or concomitant to it.

Clinical management

There are no protocols for the treatment of dogs and cats with $CvRD_{CK}$. In any case, it should be individualised based on the clinical signs and diagnostic findings. However, it is clear that treatment for CKD should be initiated. Its aim is to delay disease progression and achieve a better patient quality of life. Early diagnosis is therefore important, because the earlier treatment starts, the greater the chance of obtaining positive results and for a longer period of time. As CKD develops, side effects on other organs, amongst which the cardiovascular system is particularly important, also become more apparent.

It is very important to try to identify the causes responsible for the disease. For example, in the Mediterranean basin, a common cause of CKD is canine leishmaniasis. In these cases, specific treatment against the parasitic disease is a priority because, while it is true that the animal's CKD will not be cured, its signs will improve and the efforts made to treat it will be more successful.

In order to prevent or, if already established, treat the consequences on cardiovascular function, patient monitoring is required, with special attention to blood pressure, hydration status, blood electrolyte concentration, level of uraemia, severity of anaemia, and supervision of the medication administered (renally excreted drugs should be avoided, especially those prescribed for heart diseases). It is very important to define the level of disease severity, for which the IRIS classification is very useful.

It should be attempted to maintain systolic blood pressure below 160 mmHg. In addition to the start of treatment with antihypertensive drugs, a specific diet for renal disease is very helpful. Blood pressure monitoring should include normotensive patients. Hydration status also needs to be monitored. For long periods of time the animal maintains water balance, unless the animal does not have free access to drinking water. This balance may be impaired during uraemic crises, which are associated with persistent vomiting and depression, leading the animal to decreased water intake while remaining polyuric. By contrast, in end stages with oliguria/anuria, the most serious risk is development of hyperhydration secondary to fluid therapy.

On the other hand, chronic cardiac dysfunction itself, once established, requires follow-up with chest X-rays, echocardiography and, if possible, blood biomarkers to help assess cardiovascular impairment.

Information from human medicine suggests that patients may achieve a balance and control of renal and cardiac dysfunction over a variable period of time. Veterinary research will probably establish the diagnostic protocols to be used in these cases in the near future.

05

CARDIOVASCULAR–RENAL DISORDERS SECONDARY TO SYSTEMIC DISEASES AND CONCOMITANT CARDIORENAL DISEASES

Domingo Casamián-Sorrosal

Introduction

Cardiorenal syndrome (CRS) type 5 or $CvRD_0$ includes systemic diseases that lead to simultaneous damage or dysfunction of the kidney and cardiovascular system (Pouchelon et al., 2015; Ronco et al., 2009). This classification also usually includes patients in whom independent renal and cardiac disease (e.g. primary glomerular disease and mitral valve disease) occur simultaneously (Pouchelon et al., 2015).

In general, the coexistence of and relationship between renal disease and cardiac disease in these patients will have the same points of pathophysiological interaction described in depth for the other types of CRS (Fig. 1), though the specific mechanisms of damage and cardiac and renal dysfunction of each primary disease would be added to these. General factors leading to CRS include activation of the sympathetic nervous system and the renin–angiotensin–aldosterone system (RAAS), anaemia, oxidative stress, cell apoptosis and fibrosis, decreased cardiac output, cardiac and vascular remodelling, increased intraglomerular pressure, decreased renal perfusion and glomerular filtration rate, venous congestion, peripheral vasoconstriction, and systemic arterial hypertension (Ronco et al., 2008a).

Many conditions can lead to renal and cardiovascular damage or dysfunction, but include the following: sepsis or systemic inflammatory response syndrome (SIRS), certain infectious diseases, certain toxic substances, embolic disease (septic, neoplastic or thrombotic), gastric dilatation-volvulus, certain infiltrative diseases (e.g. amyloidosis or lysosomal diseases), and some endocrine diseases (e.g. hyperadrenocorticism, diabetes or hyperthyroidism) (Pouchelon et al., 2015; Ronco et al., 2009; Ronco et al., 2008b). Depending on the type of condition, cardiovascular and renal damage and dysfunction will be either acute (e.g. sepsis or embolism) or chronic (e.g. endocrine diseases).

Diagnosis

In general, the same diagnostic tools as described in the previous chapters are used for the other types of CRS; however, some of these tests may also be affected by primary disease, which in many cases is initially unknown.

Assessment of heart damage

In general, the **physical examination** will be poorly specific, but may lead to suspected heart disease. Findings that may indicate the presence of cardiac disease

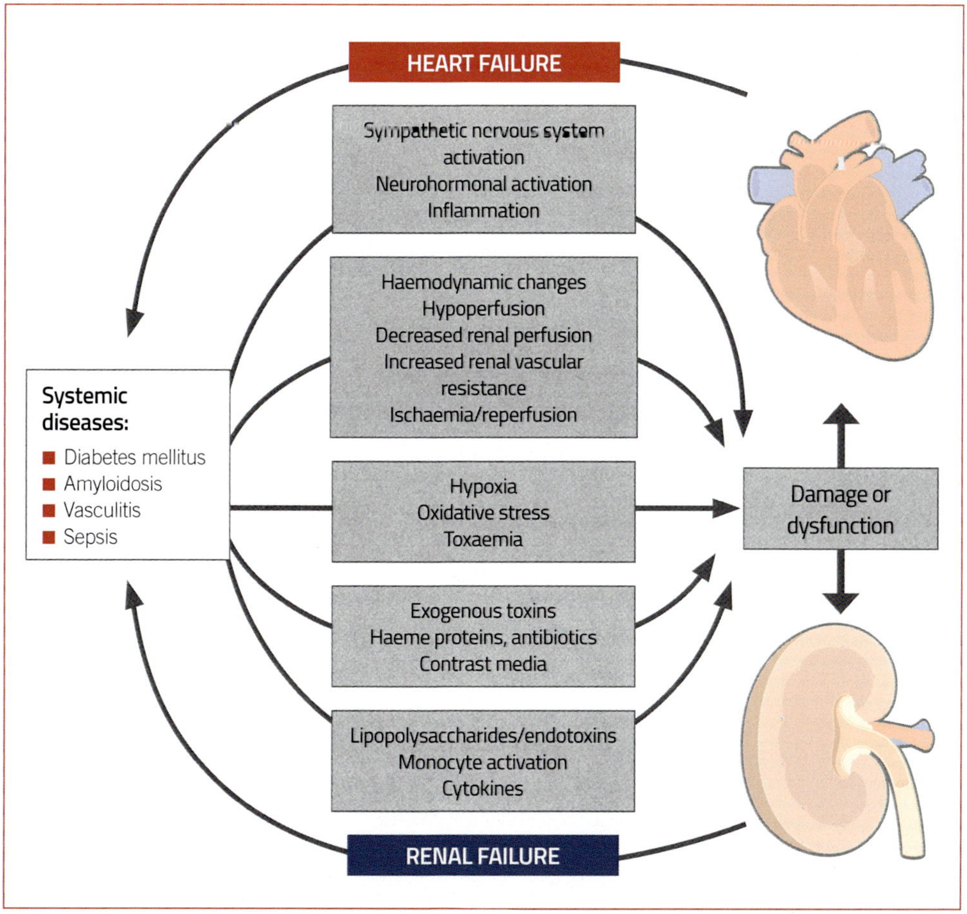

Figure 1. Pathophysiological interactions between heart and kidneys in cardiorenal syndrome type 5 (or secondary cardiorenal syndrome) (Adapted from Ronco et al., 2008a).

(e.g. murmur) may also be due to underlying primary heart disease. In addition, overlapping cases are often the most clinically significant, i.e. cases in which an underlying cardiac disease worsens or decompensates due to systemic disease.

The presence of clinical signs of shock or circulatory collapse (pale mucous membranes, prolonged capillary refill time, low temperature, weak pulses) may be due to cardiogenic shock, as well as to other types of shock caused by the underlying disease. In general, the clinician must be aware during the treatment or diagnostic procedure of a systemic disease that the decrease in blood pressure may be caused (at least in part) by a decrease in cardiac output. A patient with right congestive heart failure will usually show some of the following signs: jugular distension or pulsation, ascites, tachypnoea, and attenuated cardiac sounds if there is a pleural or pericardial effusion, and more rarely peripheral oedema. However, in patients with prior systemic disease these signs may be masked and the first indication of right congestive heart failure may be an increase in central venous pressure (>10 mmHg) in patients monitored with a central venous catheter. Dogs with left congestive heart failure will always have tachypnoea and tachycardia, and cats, tachypnoea and variable heart rate. However, heart rate (and even respiratory rate) may already be impaired initially in patients with $CVRD_0$ due to the underlying disease and, therefore, the clinician should take into account that when a critically-ill patient with a systemic disease develops progressive tachypnoea with dyspnoea and a restrictive respiratory pattern, accompanied by a decrease in oxygen saturation (<95 %) or an increased alveolar-arterial gradient (>25–35 mm Hg), this may be due, among other causes, to cardiogenic pulmonary oedema.

In general, except for murmurs due to valvular endocarditis secondary to a septic process (diastolic at the base if aortic and systolic at the apex if mitral), most murmurs in cases of systemic diseases are low grade (less than 3/6) in the left base and poorly specific, since they occur very often without significant cardiac changes caused by alterations in blood properties (e.g. anaemia) or increased total plasma volume (e.g. sepsis). Many other murmurs (especially if detected at initial examination) may be due to underlying primary heart disease. The presence of diastolic sounds (gallop rhythm) is more specific, and these are often the result of diastolic dysfunction.

The presence of arrhythmias, particularly if severe, may indicate damage to or dysfunction of the heart, so specific cardiac assessment is required. Tachyarrhythmias and bradyarrhythmias may contribute to some of the clinical signs (e.g. collapse or weakness) and the observed haemodynamic changes (e.g. hypotension). If arrhythmia is suspected, an **ECG** (Fig. 2) and continuous electrocardiographic monitoring should be performed in critical cases.

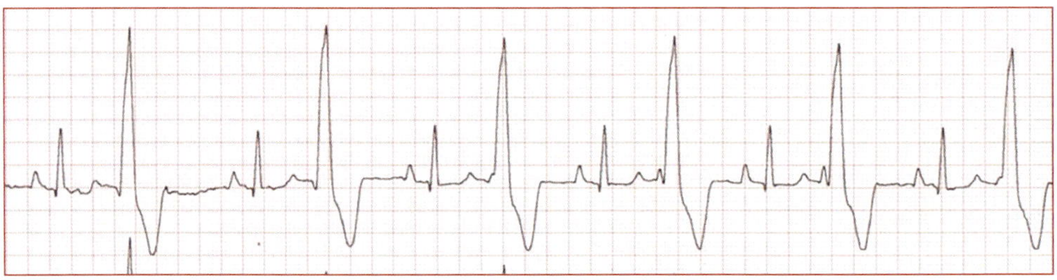

Figure 2. Electrocardiogram (lead II at 50 mm/s) from a mixed-breed dog taken during treatment of immune-mediated polyarthritis. A bigeminal rhythm is seen, with frequent ventricular premature complexes. The dog also had moderate proteinuria and increased SDMA and troponin I levels.

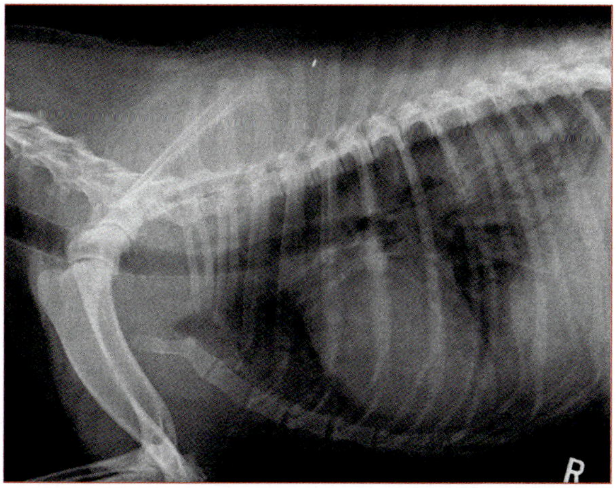

Figure 3. Lateral X-ray of a dog with bacterial endocarditis of the aortic valve, SIRS, severe renal dysfunction, and left congestive heart failure. Left heart enlargement with left atrial enlargement and an interstitial pattern progressing to an alveolar pattern in the caudodorsal lobes suggesting pulmonary oedema are seen. Pulmonary oedema was cardiogenic, but SIRS-induced pneumonitis and uraemia could also be precipitating or contributing factors.

The primary utility of **thoracic radiography** is to identify cardiomegaly and congestive heart failure. In case of left congestive heart failure, pulmonary vein distension and pulmonary oedema (often perihilar in dogs and multifocal in cats) will be observed (Fig. 3). However, it is very important to keep in mind that many of the diseases encompassed within $CvRD_0$ may be associated with pulmonary infiltrates, either due to noncardiogenic oedema, pneumonitis, pneumonia or infiltrates secondary to pulmonary thromboembolism.

Thoracic ultrasound is useful for identifying pulmonary changes such as pulmonary oedema (mainly the presence of B-lines). However, these will be poorly specific and, as in X-rays, may be caused by other changes in the lung parenchyma due to the underlying disease. Pleural effusion, ascites, or hepatic congestion may also be detected in the case of right heart failure.

Echocardiography is the most useful diagnostic tool for evaluating both possible underlying primary heart disease and structural and functional alterations caused by systemic disease (Fig. 4). There are five aspects to be considered in patients in whom a secondary CRS is suspected:

- The presence or absence of eccentric (enlargement) or concentric cardiac hypertrophy
- Structural and echogenicity changes both in the valves and in the atrial and ventricular walls
- Systolic function
- Diastolic function and ventricular filling pressures
- The presence of "intracavitary echocardiographic smoke" or vascular or intracardiac thrombi

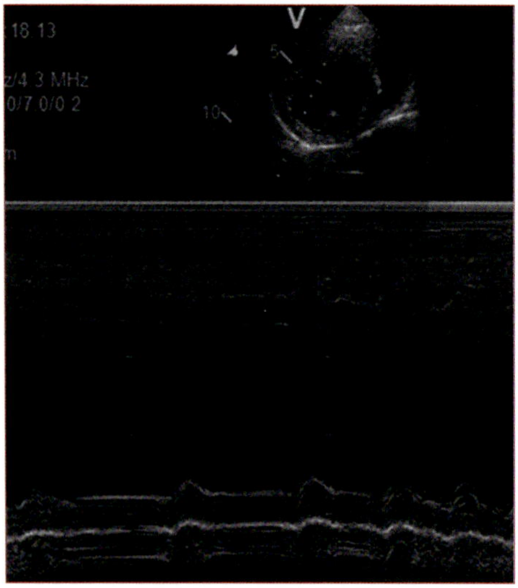

Figure 4. Transthoracic echocardiography of a dog with severe hypothyroidism (the patient had deep lethargy, bradycardia and weakness of the posterior third). M-mode performed on the short axis at the papillary muscles level (just below the mitral valve). Mild to moderate systolic dysfunction is seen, with alteration of all systolic parameters. There is an increase in the ventricular systolic dimension and a decreased shortening fraction (18 %). Heart rate and echocardiographic changes returned to normal after treatment (in a 5-month follow-up echocardiogram).

Assessment of systolic and diastolic function may be done using basic ultrasound and more advanced techniques such as conventional tissue Doppler, deformation (strain) analysis or speckle-tracking. In addition, considering the invasive (and costly in some cases) nature of techniques such as thermodilution and lithium dilution, ultrasound is the main practical method for determining cardiac output in daily clinical practice. Many systemic diseases are associated with echocardiographic changes (Table 1), and the clinician must interpret in each patient if these changes are slight and not clinically significant (which occurs very often), or if they have a haemodynamic and clinical impact on the patient.

The most important **cardiac biomarkers** are the N-terminal pro–B-type natriuretic peptide (NT-proBNP) (Oyama et al., 2013) and cardiac troponin I (cTnI) (Fonfara et al., 2010). The NT-proBNP is the most commonly used natriuretic peptide and is derived from the protein (and intracellular precursor of B-type natriuretic peptide) proBNP (Winter et al., 2017). It is synthesised in myocytes stimulated by an acute or chronic increase in ventricular stress (Oyama et al., 2013). The NT-proBNP peptide has been shown to be a useful tool in the diagnosis of certain primary heart diseases, particularly for the diagnosis of heart failure in patients with dyspnoea (Oyama et al., 2013). Natriuretic peptides are also elevated in many extracardiac diseases including: various metabolic diseases, renal disease, systemic hypertension, pulmonary hypertension, anaemia, or various cancers (Kellihan et al., 2011; Lalor et al., 2009; Menaut et al., 2012; Pelander et al., 2017; Raffan et al., 2009). However, their determination in daily clinical practice to detect cardiac dysfunction in the course of a systemic disease is, with the information available today, questionable. Their elevation is influenced, for example, by the volaemic state, afterload (e.g. arterial vasoconstriction) or the presence of pulmonary hypertension. Perhaps their most promising future use could be to help rule out cardiogenic heart failure (when values are normal) or as prognostic factors. Further studies in specific clinical situations are needed to establish their clinical use in $CvRD_0$.

Table 1. Echocardiographic changes that may be observed in some of the disease conditions occurring in secondary cardiorenal syndrome.

Disease	Echocardiographic changes
Sepsis, SIRS (described in dogs, although similar changes are usually seen in cats)	■ Enlarged cardiac chambers ■ Systolic and diastolic dysfunction ■ Slight regurgitation (mitral, tricuspid). Generally increased cardiac output (but may vary depending on blood volume)
Acromegaly (cat)	■ Left ventricular hypertrophy ■ Diastolic dysfunction ■ Enlarged left atrium
Anaemia (dog and cat: findings, particularly cardiac dimensions, vary from hypovolaemic, normovolaemic, or hypervolaemic anaemia)	■ Increased heartbeat volume (volume per beat) and cardiac output ■ Decreased left ventricular systolic dimensions and E-point septal separation ■ Increased shortening fraction ■ Variable atrial and ventricular diastolic dimensions depending on volume level
Diabetes mellitus (dog and cat)	■ Slightly increased or normal systolic and diastolic ventricular dimensions ■ Diastolic dysfunction
Hyperthyroidism (cat)	■ Atrial enlargement (unilateral or bilateral) ■ Concentric or eccentric ventricular hypertrophy ■ Diastolic dysfunction (rarely systolic) ■ Ventricular outlet tract obstructions
Hypothyroidism (dog)	■ Decreased left ventricular free wall and interventricular septum thickness ■ Systolic dysfunction ■ Decreased shortening fraction ■ Increased left ventricular end-systolic dimension
Hyperadrenocorticism (dog)	■ Left ventricular hypertrophy ■ Increased ventricular mass index
Systemic hypertension (dogs and cats)	■ Concentric left ventricular hypertrophy

Taken from: Acierno et al., 2018; Bond et al., 1988; Bulmer, 2011; Chetboul et al., 2003; Cortadellas et al., 2006; Dickinson et al., 2007; Kim et al., 2018; Little and Gettinby, 2008; Myers et al., 2014; Nelson and Thompson, 2006; Panciera, 1994; Pereira et al., 2017; Syme, 2007; Takano et al., 2015.

Troponin I is a regulatory protein of the cardiac muscle contractile apparatus. It is an escape marker: damage to the integrity of the membrane of cardiac myocytes results in its release into the blood. Minor (and in many cases reversible) cell damage will result in cytosolic troponin release (2–4 % of total troponin), while severe (and usually irreversible) cell damage will result in structural troponin release (Wells and Sleeper, 2008). The number of damaged cells (and not only the severity of this damage) and the time elapsed between myocardial damage and sample collection will also influence troponin levels (Wells and Sleeper, 2008). In general, troponin I is a marker of myocardial damage, not function, though logically both are related. Increases in troponin I have been documented during numerous extracardiac systemic conditions, including babesiosis, ehrlichiosis, leishmaniosis, parvovirosis, leptospirosis, sepsis, endotoxemia, SIRS, gastric dilatation-volvulus, severe respiratory disease, pulmonary hypertension, renal disease, immune-mediated haemolytic anaemia, seizures, pancreatitis, or neoplasms (lymphoma, visceral neoplasm) (Diniz et al., 2008; Dutton et al., 2017; Gow et al., 2011; Guglielmini et al., 2010; Hamacher et al., 2015; Langhorn and Willesen, 2015; Lobetti et al., 2002; Martínez-Hernández et al., 2017; Schober et al., 2002; Serra et al., 2010; Sharkey et al., 2009). Moreover, troponin I correlates with disease severity or is a prognostic factor in SIRS (Hamacher et al., 2015), babesiosis (Lobetti et al., 2002), leishmaniosis (Martínez-Hernández et al., 2017), parvovirosis (Kocaturk et al., 2012), gastric dilatation-volvulus (Schober et al., 2002) and generally in cases of dogs with a critical illness with systemic inflammation (Langhorn et al., 2014).

In patients with $CvRD_O$, it is also important to evaluate **cardiovascular function as a whole,** taking into account the interrelationship between the heart, vascular system and kidney. Moreover, many of the underlying diseases associated with secondary CRS cause multiple organ dysfunction syndrome (MODS). To assess cardiovascular function globally (including, in addition to heart function, vascular tone and blood volume), basic physical examination parameters such as mucous membrane colour and capillary refill time, presence of clinical dehydration, heart rate and, particularly, as an overall value, blood pressure are normally used. Detection of tissue hypoxia (imbalance between oxygen consumption and distribution), which may be abnormal even with normal cardiac output and blood pressure, can be clinically evaluated by measuring lactate, base deficit, and central venous oxygen saturation (Conti-Patara et al., 2012).

Assessment of kidney damage

Clinically, renal dysfunction will cause general signs (e.g. lethargy, vomiting) that are not specific and will often overlap with the underlying disease during $CvRD_O$. The presence of anuria, oliguria, or polyuria is more specific and may alert to renal dysfunction in the course of a systemic disease. In the laboratory setting, measurement or estimation of glomerular filtration rate (GFR), glomerular damage and tubular damage is the cornerstone of kidney damage assessment. Although GFR (typically 4.5 ml/min/kg in dogs and 2.5–3.5 ml/min/kg in cats) can be calculated directly using plasma creatinine or iohexol clearance, or radioisotope scans, the most common method of estimating GFR is by measuring plasma creatinine concentration (and, to a lesser extent, SDMA). Measurement of creatinine is the initial method of this assessment of both chronic and acute renal diseases (see tables on pages 41 and 72). Assessment of the urine protein:creatinine ratio, urinary concentration in relation to blood volume, and presence of glycosuria, haematuria, pyuria, or granular or cellular casts also provide information on possible renal impairment. Certain urinary enzymes, such as γ-glutamyl transferase (GGT), cauxin or neutrophil gelatinase-associated lipocalin (NGAL) (Orvalho and Cowgill, 2017), are promising markers of tubular damage that can detect renal disease (acute or chronic) before the development of azotaemia. Their use is not yet standardised in daily clinical practice.

Renal ultrasound and computed tomography (CT) may also provide useful information to diagnose or rule out some systemic conditions.

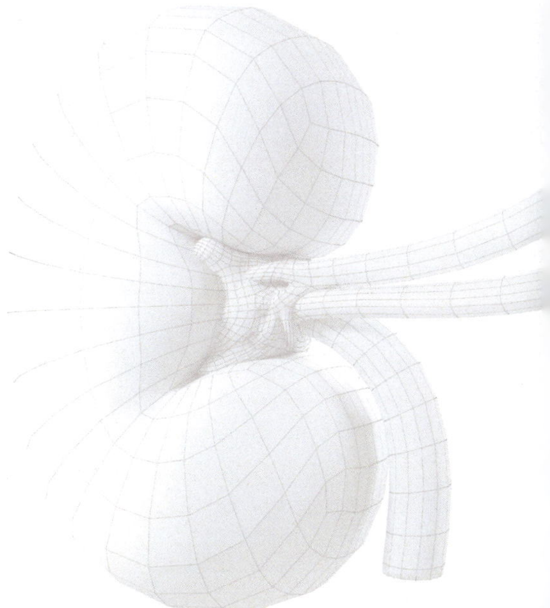

Critical patients: sepsis, SIRS, shock, and infectious diseases

Many of these patients have different degrees of cardiac and renal dysfunction, from mild (with cTnI <1 ng/ml) to severe (with cTnI >10 ng/ml) (Langhorn and Willesen, 2015). The pathogenesis of cardiac dysfunction in these patients is multifactorial and complex (Box 1). Myocardial involvement with ventricular dilation and systolic and diastolic dysfunction are common in septic patients with SIRS, and should be taken into account because they may be causes or factors involved in hypotension and pulmonary oedema (Bulmer, 2011). This dysfunction is usually reversible (Bulmer, 2011; Langhorn and Willesen, 2015). Various cytokines (TNF-α, IL-6, IL-1, IL-8, IL-10, and IL-15) play an important role in myocardial injury and dysfunction in these cases. Kidney injury in sepsis occurs, in addition to hypoperfusion, due to inflammation that causes tubular damage and generalised oxidative damage (Keir and Kellum, 2015). It should also be noted that many of these patients suffer from multiple organ dysfunction syndrome (MODS). The clinical management of patients with $CvRD_O$ should be individualised to achieve a clinical balance (Fig. 5). As explained in previous chapters, management of CRS in general should consist in maintaining good renal perfusion with adequate urine production; avoiding renal venous congestion; avoiding nephrotoxic treatments; maintaining adequate blood pressure (mean above 65 mmHg) without increasing central venous pressure using adequate fluid therapy (with caution to avoid

Box 1. Factors or causes (initiating or contributing) of secondary myocardial damage in the course of systemic or metabolic diseases (taken from Langhorn and Willesen, 2015).

- Hypotension
- Hypoxaemia
- Anaemia
- Fever
- Tachycardia
- Increased myocardial wall stress
- Arrhythmia
- Endothelial/microvascular dysfunction
- Microthrombosis
- Pulmonary thromboembolism
- Toxic effects of endotoxins
- Toxic effects of inflammatory cytokines
- Oxidative stress
- Epicardial and endocardial haemorrhage
- Reperfusion injury following stabilisation procedures
- Inotropic and vasopressor drugs
- Cardiotoxic drugs (e.g. doxorubicin)
- Poisoning by arthropod or ophidian venom

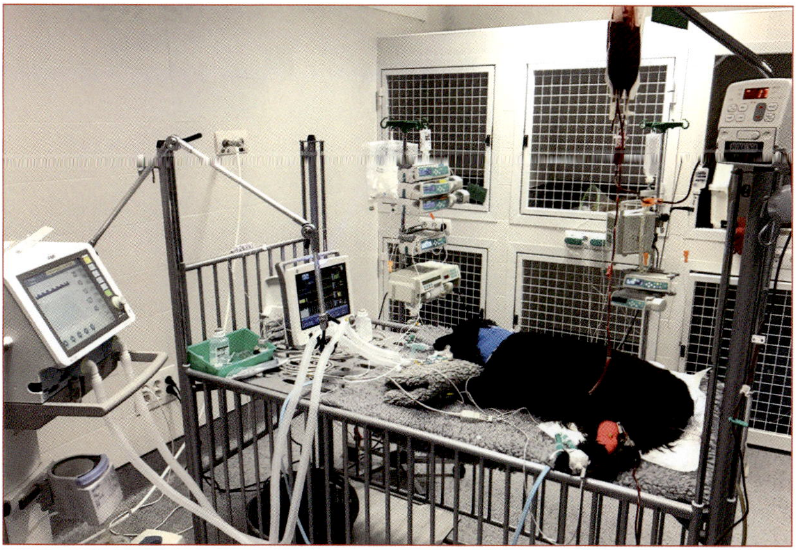

Figure 5. Intensive care of a critically ill dog with myocardial injury (arrhythmia), pulmonary oedema and renal failure, among other disorders. The patient is receiving oxygen therapy, a blood transfusion, and has pressure and urine output monitoring by arterial, central venous and urinary catheterisation. Image courtesy of Vicente Herrería (Head of Intensive Care Unit, Veterinary Teaching Hospital, Catholic University of Valencia).

pulmonary oedema) and, in some cases, with administration of vasopressors or positive inotropes; and monitoring and treating arrhythmias, if haemodynamically significant. The important thing in this type of CRS will also be to implement intensive, urgent treatment (the latter especially in the case of bacterial sepsis – Keir and Kellum, 2015) against the underlying cause.

Endocrine diseases

Diabetes mellitus

Both canine and feline patients with diabetes mellitus have diastolic dysfunction that appears to progress as the disease progresses (Kim et al., 2018; Pereira et al., 2017). It is important to keep this in mind, particularly in critically ill patients (e.g. in a ketoacidotic crisis) who may require intensive fluid therapy or in those patients with underlying heart disease, since they will be at a higher risk of developing congestive heart failure. In this setting, one study suggested that the prevalence of heart failure in cats with diabetes mellitus is greater than in similar-aged cats without diabetes mellitus (Little and Gettinby, 2008).

These patients could also have cardiovascular autonomic neuropathy, of which there is evidence in dogs (Kenefick et al., 2007). Although diabetic nephropathy (with glomerular lesions causing proteinuria and tubular damage) has been reported in dogs and cats, its clinical significance is unknown due to overlap with idiopathic renal disease.

Hyperthyroidism

Thyroid hormones regulate cardiac function through isoformic changes of myosin, the activity of sarcoplasmic reticulum Ca^{2+}-ATPase of and other ion transporters and also because of their influence on the number of β-adrenergic receptors (Bond et al., 1988).

In hyperthyroidism, there is also usually an increase in cardiac output due to increased systolic function and peripheral vasodilation due to increased metabolism (Fine et al., 2010; Sangster et al., 2013). Hyperthyroid cardiomyopathy is heterogeneous in presentation, and various remodelling processes may be seen on echocardiography (Table 1). Alterations are suspected to depend on the severity and duration of the hyperthyroid state. If these are mild, or even moderate, they can revert to normal after treatment. The presence of heart failure is more abnormal today, as the disease is detected earlier (Syme, 2007). Many hyperthyroid cats suffer occult CKD that may become evident when treating hyperthyroidism, as treatment for hyperthyroidism decreases GFR by decreasing renal perfusion (Syme, 2007).

Hypothyroidism

Cardiovascular physical findings include bradycardia or decreased heartbeat intensity. Electrocardiographic changes include sinus bradycardia, decreased amplitude of P and R waves, and first- and second-degree atrioventricular block (Beier et al., 2014). Although they may be present and must be considered, particularly in patients with underlying heart disease, arrhythmias and myocardial dysfunction (Table 1 and Fig. 4) are not significant in most hypothyroid dogs and disappear once euthyroid status is achieved with treatment (Beier et al., 2014).

06

ANAESTHETIC MANAGEMENT OF PATIENTS WITH CARDIOVASCULAR–RENAL AXIS DISORDERS

Fernando Martínez Taboada

Introduction

Patients with cardiovascular–renal disorders are an anaesthetic challenge. The risk/benefit of the procedure to be performed must always be weighed, if it is necessary, and if it is routine (and can wait for stabilisation).

Most of these patients are usually classified as ASA (American Society of Anesthesiologists) categories 2 to 5, and it should be taken into account that anaesthetic morbidity and mortality increase with ASA classification (Table 1). Redondo (2018) recently reported the latest perianaesthetic mortality data in Spain, and found ASA categories 3 to 5 and cachexia to be predictors of mortality when compared to healthy patients (ASA 1) and those with a normal body mass.

Depending on the severity of the cardiorenal disorders, the pharmacokinetics and pharmacodynamics of the anaesthetic drugs will also be more or less altered. Cachexia, as well as dehydration and oedema formation, alter the volume of distribution of drugs. The decrease in cardiac output and peripheral perfusion reduces the absorption of drugs administered intramuscularly or subcutaneously. Decreased cardiac output also alters the distribution time of the drugs and the effect on the target organs (e.g. increased arm–brain time, but more rapid changes in anaesthetic depth). Many patients with cardiovascular–renal disorders

Table 1. ASA (American Society of Anesthesiologists) classification of anaesthetic risk.

ASA category	Physical description	Examples
1	A healthy patient or with a minor, well located problem.	■ Castrations ■ Skin suture
2	Patient with mild systemic disease without functional limitations.	■ Skin tumour ■ Fracture without shock ■ Compensated heart disease ■ Compensated diabetes
3	Patient with severe systemic disease.	■ Azotaemia ■ Decompensated diabetes ■ Decompensated heart disease ■ Severe dehydration
4	Patient with severe systemic disease that is a constant threat to life.	■ Sepsis ■ Decompensated heart failure
5	A moribund patient who is not likely to survive 24 hours without the procedure.	■ Extreme shock ■ Extreme trauma ■ Multiple organ failure
E	Patient who requires emergency surgery (must be added to one of the above categories).	■ Haemoabdomen ■ Gastric volvulus

also have hypoproteinaemia, which causes the unbound fraction of any drug to be increased. Therefore, the therapeutic response to a given dose of a highly protein-bound drug (e.g. propofol, lidocaine) is greater. Decreased hepatic and renal perfusion have a direct effect on drug metabolism and elimination, increasing the duration of the effect.

Virtually all drugs used in anaesthesia (with the exception of ketamine) cause a blockade of sympathetic tone and a decrease in cardiac contractility and rate, which can range from negligible (e.g. diazepam, midazolam) to severe (e.g. medetomidine, dexmedetomidine). These pharmacological effects should be taken into account when designing an anaesthetic protocol for a specific patient.

Finally, most drugs used to treat these disorders interact with anaesthetics, which makes the dose–effect response of the latter difficult to predict.

Patients with cardiovascular disease affecting the renal system

Heart diseases have specific pathophysiologies which vary greatly from one to another. In addition, the disease may be more or less compensated and the severity of clinical signs may vary. Therefore, clinicians should try not to encompass all heart diseases in the same group.

The goal of the anaesthetic protocol should be to prevent worsening of cardiac function, increased myocardial work, and therefore metabolic oxygen consumption (MO_2C). MO_2C depends on heart rate, contractility, afterload (peripheral vascular resistance), and myocardial wall tension. It should also be taken into account that myocardial perfusion (*Q*M) occurs during diastole and is dependent on diastolic blood pressure (DBP) and left ventricular end-diastolic pressure (LVEDP).

$$QM = \frac{(\text{DBP} - \text{LVEDP})}{\text{Myocardial vascular resistance}}$$

As much clinical information about the patient as possible should be obtained. Echocardiography will allow an accurate diagnosis to be made, and the severity of the animal's heart disease to be assessed. In cases where there is left heart compromise or dyspnoea, it is advisable to obtain chest X-rays to evaluate, among other things, the presence of pulmonary oedema or pulmonary disease. An electrocardiogram (ECG) may be very useful when arrhythmias are suspected. Patient evaluation should include functionality of other organs such as the kidney and liver, as well as assessment of the acid–base balance and electrolyte levels.

Whenever the procedure can be scheduled, it is advisable to evaluate the heart medication given to the patient, to know its effects on the anaesthetic and analgesic drugs, and to decide when the medication should be discontinued before anaesthesia (Table 2).

Acute cardiovascular disorders

Heart failure syndrome is a ventricular dysfunction characterised by a cardiac output lower than the metabolic demands of the body. After a complete physical examination (including blood pressure measurement, peripheral temperature assessed by touch and haematological, electrolyte and blood biochemistry) and analysis of the medical history and current treatment, it should be established whether the patient can be anaesthetised safely or requires prior stabilisation. In general, if dyspnoea, cyanosis, tachycardia, and marked exercise intolerance are present, the patient is unlikely to survive the anaesthetic period (Fig. 1).

Decision-making to determine whether a heart patient can be anaesthetised or not is based on several pillars:

1. Prior cardiovascular assessment and changes since last assessment.

Table 2. Therapeutic effect of the most common cardiac medications and potential interactions with anaesthetic agents (adapted from Rioja et al., 2016).

Cardiac medication	Therapeutic effect	Possible adverse effect during anaesthesia
ACEIs (enalapril, benacepril)	Peripheral vasodilation.	Hypotension
Digoxin	Increases contractility and decreases heart rate.	Bradycardia
Phosphodiesterase Inhibitors and calcium sensitizers (pimobendan)	Increase myocardial contractility and cause peripheral vasodilation.	Hypotension
Calcium channel blockers (diltiacem)	Decrease ventricular sensitivity to supraventricular tachycardia, promote myocardial relaxation, and cause arterial vasodilation.	■ Hypotension. Enhancement of the effect of neuromuscular blocking agents
β- adrenergic blockers (propranolol, atenolol)	Decrease heart rate, contractility and conductivity.	■ Bradycardia ■ Hypotension ■ Cardiac blocks
Diuretics (furosemide, spironolactone)	Eliminate retained excess fluid and sodium (oedema) and reduce preload.	Hypotension

Author's recommendation: Angiotensin-converting enzyme inhibitor (ACEI) therapy should be discontinued 2 days before anaesthesia if possible and calcium channel inhibitors should be discontinued 24 hours before anaesthesia. These drugs are most likely to interact with anaesthetics, and very severe cases of hypotension may be seen. If the patient is receiving diuretics, volume and degree of dehydration (if any) should be corrected prior to anaesthetic induction.

2. The presence of certain predictors of cardiac risk (decompensated congestive heart failure, arrhythmias with haemodynamic effects, pulmonary oedema, diabetes mellitus, renal failure, hypertension, etc.).
3. Degree of exercise tolerance.
4. Risk attributable to surgery per se (anatomical location of surgery, duration, and associated bleeding) (Fig. 2).

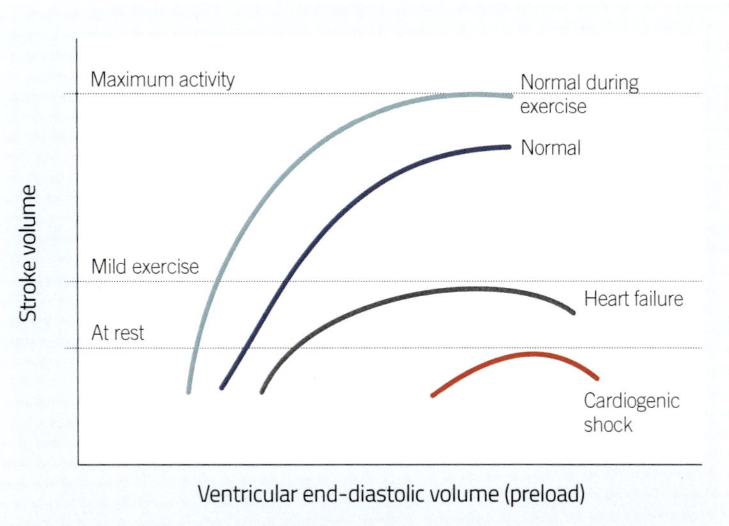

Figure 1. Frank-Starling law of the heart (adapted from Rioja et al., 2016).

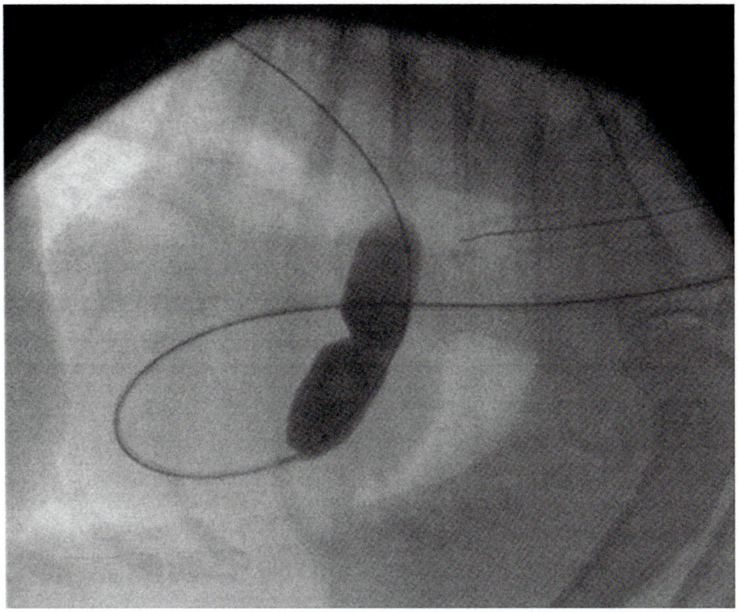

Figure 2. Balloon valvuloplasty in a case of pulmonary valve stenosis.

Assessment of these aspects will determine whether the patient can be anaesthetised with an acceptable risk or requires specific treatment (Fig. 3).

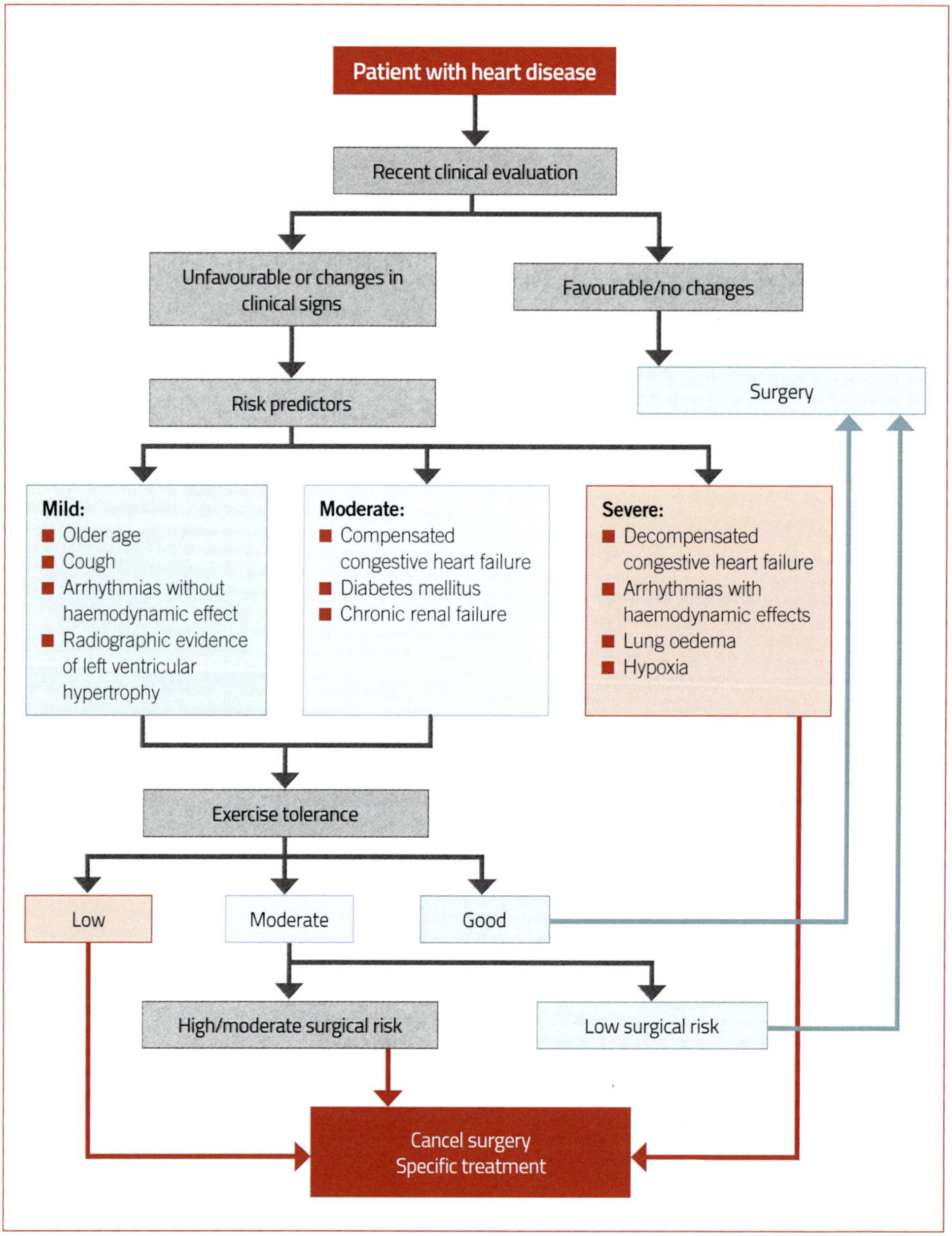

Figure 3. Decision making before the anaesthetic procedure for patients with heart disease.

In cases where the anaesthetic procedure is considered adequate, it is characterised by:

- **Preanaesthetic period and premedication.** Prior stabilisation of cardiac function (contractility and heart rhythm) and blood volume is essential. The patient's stress level should be reduced, and preoxygenation is essential provided it is tolerated. In many cases sedation/premedication is only performed with an opioid, e.g. methadone (0.2 mg/kg) or butorphanol (0.2 mg/kg). The use of benzodiazepines may be advisable, though sometimes a paradoxical excitation can be observed that could increase oxygen consumption. Because of this, the author prefers to use diazepam or midazolam as coinduction agents. If the patient requires intramuscular sedation to obtain vascular access, the use of a relatively high-dose opioid (methadone: 0.4–0.5 mg/kg) mixed with alfaxalone (1 mg/kg) is usually sufficient.
- **Induction.** The use of coinduction, understood as the combination of drugs to reduce their doses and obtain more favourable cardiopulmonary characteristics, is useful. Combinations of midazolam (0.2–0.3 mg/kg) with either alfaxalone or propofol dosed according to effect have shown high cardiovascular stability, causing very good induction and endotracheal intubation conditions. There are studies showing a greater stability of cardiac output with alfaxalone, though the effects with both drugs are very transient.
- **Monitoring.** It should be comprehensive and include ECG, blood pressure (preferably invasive), capnography, peripheral pulse oximetry, and body temperature. It should start as soon as possible and continue until the recovery period.
- **Maintenance.** All anaesthetics cause a decrease in myocardial contractility and some peripheral vasodilation. All of this may trigger hypotension, whose treatment in these patients focuses on:
  - Adjusting the anaesthetic plane.
  - Preventing any unadvisable excess fluid by using positive inotropic drugs that help in cardiac contractility.
  - Sometimes even using vasopressors to counteract peripheral vasodilation (Fig. 4).

  As regards inotropic drugs, it is advisable to continue treatment with pimobendan until the day of anaesthesia. Dobutamine as an intravenous infusion (1–10 µg/kg/min) may also be administered for its β_1 adrenergic effects. The vasopressor drug of choice is phenylephrine (infusion at a rate of 0.5–1 µg/kg/min); it should be used with caution and after confirming that there is no response to positive inotropic drugs. Dopamine has α_1 and β_1 agonist effects, which cause increased cardiac contractility and afterload.

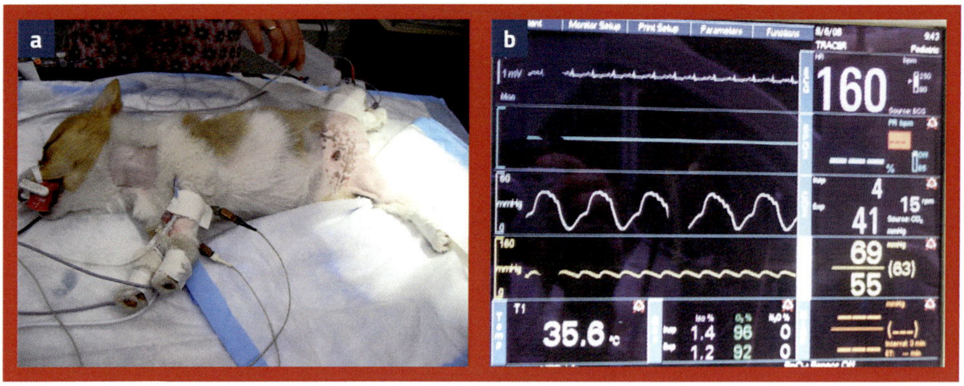

Figure 4. Dog prepared for patent ductus arteriosus embolisation using an Amplatzer device (a). Patient monitoring: relatively low pressure can be observed during the procedure (b). This procedure usually requires the use of vasopressors.

- **Analgesia.** Pain causes unwanted sympathetic stimulation in these patients. Therefore, all analgesia will be positive. The use of potent opioids is appropriate, provided they do not cause profound bradycardia affecting cardiac output. The use of regional anaesthesia is recommended, particularly epidural and spinal anaesthesia, because they cause an increase in parasympathetic tone that may be very beneficial in these patients.
- **Recovery.** Oxygenation and minimal sympathetic stimulation should be the mainstays of recovery. Therefore, the patient should be kept comfortable, normothermic, with normal blood glucose levels, free from stress, etc. Oxygen therapy is essential provided it is tolerated (e.g. oxygen therapy cages).

Chronic cardiovascular disorders

These patients are the most common in daily clinical practice. From the anaesthetic viewpoint, they can be grouped into three categories:

- Dilated cardiomyopathy and valvular insufficiency (mitral and, less commonly, tricuspid).
- Hypertrophic cardiomyopathy and valvular stenosis (pulmonary, aortic or subaortic).
- Cardiac arrhythmias (in this case the anaesthetic protocol is not considered because it exceeds the scope of the work).

Dilated cardiomyopathy and valvular insufficiency

These conditions are characterised by a more or less marked decrease in cardiac contractility depending on the severity and course of the condition. In addition, there is retrograde blood flow (regurgitation) resulting in dilatation of the right atrium for the tricuspid valve and the left atrium for the mitral valve. In general, the presence of sinus arrhythmia and low or medium heart rate during physical examination are positive signs, as well as high or moderate exercise tolerance. The purpose of the anaesthetic protocol should be:

- To maintain a moderate or high heart rate that reduces stroke time (during which regurgitation occurs).

- To promote vasodilation (to enhance antegrade versus retrograde flow).
- To optimise myocardial contractility.

The characteristics of the different phases of the anaesthetic procedure will be:

- **Premedication.** Sedation based on neuroleptoanalgesia is highly recommended. Acepromazine (0.01–0.03 mg/kg) causes a moderate degree of sedation when mixed with an opioid such as methadone (0.2 mg/kg) or butorphanol (0.2 mg/kg). Vasodilation obtained by acepromazine promotes antegrade flow. In patients requiring a greater degree of sedation, this can be obtained by adding midazolam (0.3 mg/kg), ketamine (0.5–1 mg/kg), or medetomidine (5–10 µg/kg) to the above combination. The selection of drugs will depend on the degree of sedation required, the disease and its severity. The author usually uses the combination acepromazine (0.02 mg/kg), methadone (0.2 mg/kg), and medetomidine (5 µg/kg), because it usually maintains blood pressure in a more normal range, with medetomidine counteracting the vasodilatory effects of acepromazine (Saporano et al., 2013).
- **Induction.** Depending on the severity of the condition, propofol or alfaxalone may be used (alfaxalone appears to maintain the most stable cardiac output during induction). Coinduction is also an appropriate option, combining propofol or alfaxalone with lidocaine, ketamine or benzodiazepines. Lidocaine (1–2 mg/kg IV before the inducing agent) has a direct negative inotropic effect, but its antiarrhythmic and cardioprotective effects make it a very attractive drug for this type of cases. The 1:1 combination of propofol and ketamine, known as ketofol, is a mixture of high cardiovascular stability and good induction quality in dogs, and therefore is also an option in these cases (Martínez-Taboada and Leece, 2014).
- **Monitoring.** Blood pressure monitoring is essential (Fig. 5). Depending on the severity of the clinical condition, this monitoring must be invasive or may be noninvasive. It is highly recommended to also monitor ECG, capnography, peripheral pulse oximetry, and body temperature.
- **Maintenance.** All anaesthetic drugs cause some peripheral vasodilation promoting antegrade flow. Volatile agents are recommended because they are very commonly used drugs and allow the anaesthetic plane to be adjusted very quickly. Perioperative fluids should be relatively restrictive; although they are not contraindicated, they should be administered carefully and should not be given in excess (2–4 ml/kg/h).

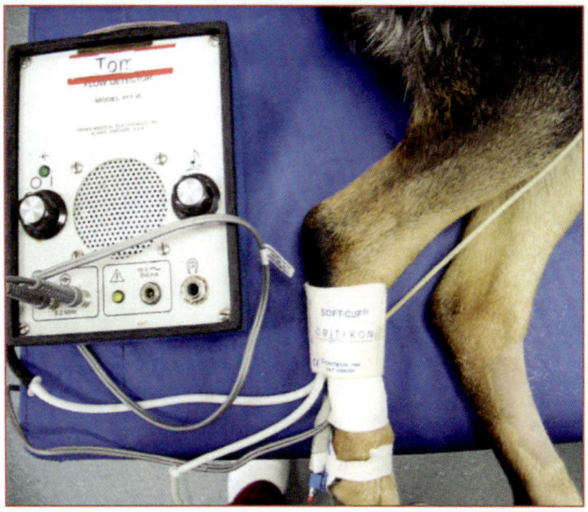

Figure 5. Measurement of blood pressure by Doppler in the perioperative period.

- **Analgesia.** Locoregional anaesthesia techniques are indicated for this type of disease to prevent excess increase in sympathetic stimulation and myocardial work. Care should be taken to maintain adequate preload (scrupulously assessing the patient's blood volume level) and to prevent bradycardia or treat it if it occurs.
- **Recovery.** Monitoring of oxygenation and cardiovascular function of the patient should continue during the postanaesthesia phase until the patient is fully recovered.

Hypertrophic cardiomyopathy and valvular stenosis

In these conditions, myocardial hypertrophy occurs primarily due to ventricular outflow tract obstruction. Thus, the following are seen:

- Increased muscle mass
- Decreased stroke volume
- Increased intracavitary pressure with decreased ventricular distensibility or compliance (large pressures are required for small volume changes)
- Increased transmural pressure
- Elongation of the isovolumetric contraction phase

The decrease in ventricular compliance determines that filling during diastole will depend on the maintenance of sinus rhythm with coordinated atrial contraction (atrial contraction accounts for 40 % of ventricular filling) and of the patient's preload (and consequently blood volume). These patients are at high risk of developing myocardial ischaemia (usually seen as ventricular arrhythmias) due to increased oxygen consumption resulting from muscle hypertrophy and elongation of the isovolumetric contraction phase, decreased oxygen supply due to diastolic shortening (coronary perfusion phase), and decreased coronary perfusion pressure (as intracavitary pressure is increased). In these patients the stroke volume is fixed, so cardiac output will mainly depend on heart rate. The objective of the anaesthetic protocol in these cases will be:

- To maintain sinus rhythm to favour ventricular filling.
- To optimise blood volume also to facilitate ventricular filling.
- To prevent profound bradycardia so that cardiac output is not severely affected.
- To prevent tachycardia that may cause increased myocardial oxygen consumption and lack of perfusion due to shortening of diastolic time.
- To prevent hypotension and vasodilation to maintain coronary preload and perfusion.

The characteristics of the different phases of the anaesthetic procedure will be:

- **Premedication.** In these patients it is highly recommended to reduce stress and its negative effects on oxygen demand and tachycardia. Preoxygenation is also recommended, but provided it is tolerated. Drugs administered should control or decrease heart rate and prevent hypotension, so the author recommends the use of α_2 adrenergic agonists such as medetomidine (5 µg/kg) in combination with an opioid such as methadone (0.2 mg/kg). It is advisable to use the intramuscular route, if possible, to prevent acute bradycardia that may seriously affect cardiac output.
- **Induction.** Once again, the goal is to keep the heart rate in a narrow range (e.g. 60–90 bpm in dogs and 100–120 bpm in cats). This can be accomplished by using alfaxalone dosed according to effect or coinduction with alfaxalone and midazolam (0.3 mg/kg), propofol with midazolam (0.3 mg/kg), or ketamine and propofol (ketofol) dosed according to effect. Propofol alone is not recommended because, when combined with medetomidine, it could trigger bradycardia affecting cardiac output. The use of ketamine alone or in combination with a benzodiazepine is also not recommended, since it may cause an excessive sympathetic stimulation that triggers an increase in heart rate and, therefore, myocardial ischaemia.
- **Monitoring.** Early ECG monitoring is recommended, as well as blood pressure control. Pulse oximetry is a good noninvasive way to monitor patient oxygenation. As in previous diseases, capnography allows simultaneous assessment of the cardiovascular and respiratory systems.
- **Maintenance.** Halogenated agents are usually those chosen for maintenance because the anaesthetic depth can be easily assessed and adjusted. Both isoflurane and sevoflurane produce dose-dependent vasodilation. Therefore, it is advisable to maintain a light anaesthetic plane and use drugs that reduce the requirements of anaesthetics, for instance, a continuous infusion of medetomidine (2–5 µg/kg/h) or dexmedetomidine (1–3 µg/kg/h).
- **Analgesia.** Continuous infusions are recommended to decrease anaesthetic requirements or sympathetic tone. The author prefers to use α_2-adrenergic agonists or lidocaine (1.8–3 mg/kg/h) to prevent an excessively low heart rate. Locoregional techniques are also recommended.
- **Recovery.** Optimisation of heart rate and preload should continue during recovery. For this, monitoring should be maintained and, if necessary, the use of sedatives should be continued during this phase.

Patients with renal disease affecting the cardiovascular system

The kidneys are responsible for or contribute to multiple vital functions such as body water preservation, electrolyte management, acid–base balance, and several hormonal and neurohormonal functions. Their primary objective is to eliminate nitrogen compounds, maintaining water and sodium homeostasis. Under normal conditions, the kidneys are unable to filter proteins or polysaccharides. They are the organs with the highest blood supply in the body, receiving 15–25 % of cardiac output. Most of this cardiac output is distributed through the renal cortex. Renal perfusion is well self-regulated between a very wide range of blood pressures, approximately between a mean pressure of 50 mmHg and 150 mmHg; outside this range blood pressure should be treated with vasopressors or ACE inhibitors to ensure renal perfusion.

Renal disease may be prerenal, renal (or intrinsic), or postrenal in origin. This condition has a direct effect on the excretion of drugs from the body and their distribution. For example, the volume of distribution of drugs may be increased or decreased if fluid retention or volume depletion exists, respectively. To adjust the drug doses, the rate of creatinine clearance should be estimated. In oliguric patients, this rate may decrease to values close to 5 ml/min. If the drug to be used requires administration of a loading bolus, the patient's extracellular fluid volume should be evaluated and a decision made as follows:

- If normal, give the standard loading bolus.
- If the patient is dehydrated (extracellular volume is small), the loading dose should be reduced.
- If the patient is retaining fluids, the loading dose is increased.

When drugs with a long half-life and a wide therapeutic index are administered, it is recommended to maintain dosing and increase the interval between doses. For drugs with a narrower therapeutic window, or with a shorter half-life, dose reduction is recommended. In human medicine, there are formulas to precisely calculate the new dose based on the renal excretion of the drug and glomerular filtration rate estimated by creatinine clearance. These tools are not available for veterinary use at this time and adjustments should be made empirically.

Anaesthesia itself may increase the risk of all patients developing renal failure of varying severity. In humans, 20 % to 50 % of cases of acute kidney injury (AKI) occur in surgical patients. In addition, these patients are eight times more likely to develop chronic kidney disease if they survive the acute phase than other subpopulations. There are several risk factors associated with AKI during anaesthesia, which are divided into preoperative and intraoperative factors (Box 1).

As in cases of heart disease, it is essential to carry out a comprehensive physical examination, review the patient's medical history, and perform laboratory tests, including haematology and electrolytes.

Depending on the origin of the renal failure, its severity and the procedure to be performed (if urgent or nonurgent), stabilisation must be performed in a more or less comprehensive and rapid manner. In general, all these patients require fluid therapy of varying intensity depending on the degree of dehydration and the presence of comorbidities (e.g. heart disease). Hyperkalaemia is common in these patients and the intensity of treatment can range from fluid therapy only to administration of insulin/dextrose or salbutamol. In cases of severe hyperkalaemia or when rapid intervention is required (e.g. sedation or anaesthesia for emergency catheterisation in a case of urethral block), administration of 10 % calcium gluconate allows malignant arrhythmia to be prevented, but does not correct plasma potassium.

Box 1. Risk factors associated with renal failure during anaesthesia.

Preoperative risk factors:

- Age
- Chronic kidney disease
- Hypertension
- Diabetes mellitus
- Congestive heart failure
- Sepsis
- Ascites
- Peripheral vascular disease
- Chronic obstructive pulmonary disease

Intraoperative risk factors:

- Intraoperative hypotension
- Duration of surgery
- Intraperitoneal surgery
- Intra-abdominal hypertension
- Heart surgery
- Nephrotoxic agents (antibiotics, contrast agents, etc.)
- Packed red blood cell transfusions
- Nonrenal organ transplant
- Cardiac surgery requiring bypass (time, haemodilution, etc.)

Anaesthesia in patients with acute kidney injury

Most of these patients require stabilisation prior to anaesthesia. In general, there is a marked decrease in glomerular filtration rate and dehydration very commonly occurs, so fluid therapy is required (the composition of fluids, as well as the amount and rate will depend on the severity of dehydration and on urine production). It is highly advisable to evaluate the ECG and blood pressure during the stabilisation phase to detect the presence of arrhythmias and hypotension requiring specific treatment. The goal of anaesthesia should be to maintain an optimum perfusion and oxygenation of the kidneys, by correcting patient hydration, cardiac output, blood pressure, and anaemia if present.

The anaesthetic procedure will be as follows:

- **Premedication.** The use of opioids is recommended as part of premedication because they are drugs with a wide safety margin that provide analgesia and some sympathetic block. Most of these patients usually have a high degree of stress and sympathetic activation that may lead to a greater decrease in renal perfusion. Benzodiazepines (midazolam: 0.2–0.3 mg/kg IV or IM) also have a wide safety margin with little effect on blood pressure and renal perfusion. Dexmedetomidine (and medetomidine by extension) is considered in human medicine to be a protective drug for kidneys in both experimental settings (protection of cells in cases of ischaemia and inhibition of apoptosis induced by hypoxia) and clinical settings (reduction of the risk of AKI in heart bypass surgery). This benefit appears to be dose-dependent. Therefore, the use of continuous infusions of dexmedetomidine (1–2 µg/kg/h) may be useful from an anxiolytic and sympathetic response-blocking standpoint and also directly beneficial for the kidneys.
- **Induction.** Some studies have suggested a certain advantage of propofol over other inducers in humans. In veterinary practice, alfaxalone administered in effective doses may also be a valid alternative.
- **Monitoring.** Cardiovascular monitoring is basic in these patients. ECG, especially in cases of moderate to severe hyperkalaemia, and blood pressure are critical parameters. If the patient requires very intensive fluid therapy, monitoring of central venous pressure or plethysmographic variation derived from the pulse oximeter may be very helpful. Finally, urine production is essential in these patients, and anaesthesia/sedation should be used to place a urinary catheter for measuring urine production in ml/kg/h.

- **Maintenance.** Inhalation anaesthesia together with administration of a continuous infusion of dexmedetomidine to reduce the requirements of isoflurane is the most advisable. Theoretically, sevoflurane is contraindicated if there is an alternative, because it interacts with soda lime producing compound A. Although compound A has been shown to be nephrotoxic in rats, it appears to be poorly active in humans and no data are available on its effect in dogs and cats.
- **Analgesia.** The use of analgesics is essential in these cases. Renal perfusion should be optimised and sympathetic activation that may compromise perfusion should be avoided. Opioids and α_2 agonists are useful drugs in patients with AKI. Epidural anaesthesia in human medicine has been associated with a decrease in the risk of perioperative AKI due to sympathetic block and some local vasodilation that promotes renal perfusion. Therefore, its use could be recommended in patients with AKI requiring surgery.
- **Recovery.** Monitoring of renal function and urine production should continue during the recovery phase. Renal perfusion should be maximised by the use of fluid therapy and vasopressors. If necessary and well tolerated by the patient, oxygen may be supplemented during recovery to improve renal oxygenation.

Anaesthesia in patients with chronic kidney injury

These patients very commonly require anaesthesia or sedation. They are often geriatric animals with a limited physiological hepatic and cardiovascular reserve. As with AKI, renal compromise, the presence of concomitant diseases, and the treatments that the patient is receiving should be assessed. If the patient suffers from hypertension and is treated with angiotensin-converting enzyme inhibitors, their administration should be stopped 24–48 hours before anaesthesia and dehydration should be corrected.

The goal during anaesthesia should be to maintain perfusion and oxygenation of the kidneys. Anaesthetic management is very similar to that in patients with AKI, but it is usually rare to find electrolyte abnormalities requiring intervention. The patient's blood pressure should be carefully monitored and any hypotensive episode prevented or corrected promptly. Administration of NSAIDs is not totally contraindicated provided blood pressure is monitored and controlled. Studies have shown a clinical benefit in patients with osteoarthritis (OA) and chronic kidney disease. In a study where low dose meloxicam was administered orally to cats with OA, an improvement was seen in musculoskeletal disease and renal disease compared to the placebo group. It may therefore be considered reasonable to administer NSAIDs once the patient is monitored and during recovery.

REFERENCES

Chapter 1. Cardiorenal syndrome in human medicine

Abraham E, Singer M. Mechanisms of sepsis-induced organ dysfunction. *Crit Care Med*, 2007; 35(10):2408–2416.

Bagshaw SM, Cruz DN, Aspromonte N, et al. Epidemiology of cardio-renal syndromes: workgroup statements from the 7th ADQI Consensus Conference. *Nephrol Dial Transplant*, 2010; 25(5):1406–1416.

Bart BA, Goldsmith SR, Lee KL, et al. Ultrafiltration in decompensated heart failure with cardiorenal syndrome. *N Engl J Med*, 2012; 367(24):2296–2304.

Bellomo R, Kellum JA, Ronco C. Acute kidney injury. *Lancet*, 2012; 380(9843):756–766.

Bock JS, Gottlieb SS. Cardiorenal syndrome new perspectives. *Circulation*, 2010; 121(23):2592–2600.

Brenner BM, Cooper ME, de Zeeuw D, et al.; RENAAL Study Investigators. Effects of losartan on renal and cardiovascular outcomes in patients with type 2 diabetes and nephropathy. *N Engl J Med*, 2001; 345(12):861–869.

Chuasuwan A, Kellum JA. Cardio–renal syndrome type 3: epidemiology, pathophysiology, and treatment. *Semin Nephrol*, 2012; 32(1):31–39.

CIBIS-II. The Cardiac Insufficiency Bisoprolol Study II (CIBIS-II): a randomised trial. *Lancet*, 1999; 353(9146):9–13.

Cice G, Ferrara L, D'Andrea A, et al. Carvedilol increases two-year survivalin dialysis patients with dilated cardiomyopathy: a prospective, placebo-controlled trial. *J Am Coll Cardiol*, 2003; 41(9):1438–1444.

Coresh J, Astor B, Sarnak MJ. Evidence for increased cardiovascular disease risk in patients with chronic kidney disease. *Curr Opin Nephrol Hypertens*, 2004; 13(1):73–81.

Cruz DN, Fard A, Clementi A, et al. Role of biomarkers in the diagnosis and management of cardio-renal syndromes. *Semin Nephrol*, 2012; 32(1):79–92.

Culleton BF, Larson MG, Wilson PW, et al. Cardiovascular disease and mortality in a community-based cohort with mild renal insufficiency. *Kidney Int*, 1999; 56(6):2214–2219.

D'Agati VD, Kaskel FJ, Falk RJ. Medical Progress: focal segmental glomerulosclerosis. *N Engl J Med*, 2011; 365(25):2398–2411.

Dar O, Cowie MR. Acute heart failure in the intensive care unit: epidemiology. *Crit Care Med*, 2008; 36(1 Suppl):S3–S8.

Di Lullo L, Floccari F, Granata A, et al. Ultrasonography: Ariadne's thread in the diagnosis of the cardiorenal syndrome. *Cardiorenal Med*, 2012; 2(1):11–17.

Di Lullo L, House A, Gorini A, et al. Chronic kidney disease and cardiovascular complications. *Heart Fail Rev*, 2015; 20(3):259–272.

Dikow R, Zeier M, Ritz E. Pathophysiology of cardiovascular disease and renal failure. *Cardiol Clin*, 2005; 23(3):311–317.

Felker GM, Lee KL, Bull DA, et al.; NHLBI Heart Failure Clinical Research Network. Diuretic strategies in patients with acute decompensated heart failure. *N Engl J Med*, 2011; 364(9):797–805.

Go AS, Chertow GM, Fan D, et al. Chronic kidney disease and the risks of death, cardiovascular events, and hospitalization. *N Engl J Med*, 2004; 351(13):1296–1305.

González Maqueda I. Enfermedad cardiovascular y función renal. Mecanismos patogénicos. In: González Juanatey JR (ed.). *Riñón y enfermedad cardíaca*. Madrid: Sociedad Española de Cardiología, 2007; pp. 11–24.

Guyton AC, Coleman TG. Quantitative analysis of the pathophysiology of hypertension. *J Am Soc Nephrol*, 1999; 10(10):2248–2259.

Hatamizadeh P, Fonarow GC, Budoff MJ, et al. Cardiorenal syndrome: pathophysiology and potential targets for clinical management. *Nat Rev Nephrol*, 2013; 9(2):99–111.

Hebert K, Dias A, Delgado MC, et al. Epidemiology and survival of the five stages of chronic kidney disease in a systolic heart failure population. *Eur J Heart Fail*, 2010; 12(8):861–865.

Herzog CA, Ma JZ, Collins AJ. Poor long-term survival after acute myocardial infarction among patients on long-term dialysis. *N Engl J Med*, 1998; 339(1):799–805.

Heymes C, Bendall JK, Ratajczak P, et al. Increased myocardial NAPH oxidase activity in human heart failure. *J Am Coll Cardiol*, 2003; 41(12):2164–2171.

Hornig B, Landmesser U, Kohler C, et al. Comparative effect of ACE inhibition and angiotensin type 1 receptor antagonism on bioavailability of nitric oxide in patients with coronary artery disease: role of superoxide dismutase. *Circulation*, 2001; 103(6):799–805.

Kellum JA, Lameire N, Aspelin P, et al. KDIGO clinical practice guideline for acute kidney injury. *Kidney Int Suppl*, 2012; 2(1):1–138.

Kim S, Iwao H. Molecular and cellular mechanisms of angiotensin II-mediated cardiovascular and renal diseases. *Pharmacol Rev*, 2000; 52(1):11–34.

Kinsey GR, Li L, Okusa MD. Inflammation in acute kidney injury. *Nephron Exp Nephrol*, 2008; 109(4):e102–107.

Kinugawa S, Tsutsui H, Hayashidani S, et al. Treatment with dimethylthiourea prevents left ventricular remodeling and failure after experimental myocardial infarction in mice: role of oxidative stress. *Circ Res*, 2000; 87(5):392–398.

Lassus JP, Nieminen MS, Peuhkurinen K, et al.; FINN-AKVA study group. Markers of renal function and acute kidney injury in acute heart failure: definitions and impact on outcomes of the cardiorenal syndrome. *Eur Heart J*, 2010; 31(22):2791–2798.

Lewis EJ, Hunsicker LG, Clarke WR, et al.; Collaborative Study Group. Renoprotective effect of the angiotensin-receptor antagonist irbesartan in patients with nephropathy due to type 2 diabetes. *N Engl J Med*, 2001; 345(12):851–860.

McMurray JJ, Packer M, Desai AS, et al.; PARADIGM-HF Investigators and Committees. Angiotensin–neprilysin inhibition versus enalapril in heart failure. *N Engl J Med*, 2014; 371(11):993–1004.

Mehta RL, Kellum JA, Shah SV, et al. Acute Kidney Injury Network: report of an initiative to improve outcomes in acute kidney injury. *Crit Care*, 2007; 11(2):R31.

MERIT-HF. Effect of metoprolol CR/XL in chronic heart failure: Metoprolol CR/XL Randomised Intervention Trial in Congestive Heart Failure (MERIT-HF). *Lancet*, 1999; 353(9169):2001–2007.

Meyer TW, Hostetter TH. Uremia. *N Engl J Med*, 2007; 357(13):1316–1325.

Muntner P, He J, Astor BC, et al. Traditional and nontraditional risk factors predict coronary heart disease in chronic kidney disease: results from the atherosclerosis risk in communities study. *J Am Soc Nephrol*, 2005; 16(2):529–538.

National Heart, Lung, and Blood Institute. Nhlbi.nih.gov [homepage on the internet]. Cardio-renal connections in heart failure and cardiovascular disease. [Updated 2005 February 18; cited 2014 Oct 10] Available from: http://www.nhlbi.nih.gov/research/reports/2004-cardiorenal-hf-hd.

Packer M, Bristow MR, Cohn JN, et al. The effect of carvedilol on morbidity and mortality in patients with chronic heart failure. U.S. Carvedilol Heart Failure Study Group. *N Engl J Med*, 1996; 334(21):1349–1355.

Pfeffer MA, Braunwald E, Moyé LA, et al. Effect of captopril on mortality and morbidity in patients with left ventricular dysfunction after myocardial infarction. Results of the survival and ventricular enlargement trial. The SAVE Investigators. *N Engl J Med*, 1992; 327(10):669–677.

Pitt B, Remme W, Zannad F, et al.; Eplerenone Post–Acute Myocardial Infarction Heart Failure Efficacy and Survival Study Investigators. Eplerenone, a selective aldosterone blocker, in patients with left ventricular dysfunction after myocardial infarction. *N Engl J Med*, 2003; 348(14):1309–1321.

Prowle JR, Echeverri JE, Ligabo EV, et al. Fluid balance and acute kidney injury. *Nat Rev Nephrol*, 2010; 6(2):107–115.

Ronco C, Haapio M, House AA, et al. Cardiorenal syndrome. *J Am Coll Cardiol*, 2008; 52(19):1527–1539.

Silverberg DS, Wexler D, Blum M, et al. The use of subcutaneous erythropoietin and intravenous iron for the treatment of the anemia of severe, resistant congestive heart failure improves cardiac andrenal function and functional cardiac class, and markedly reduces hospitalizations. *J Am Coll Cardiol*, 2000; 35(7):1737–1744.

Singh K, Xiao L, Remondino A, et al. Adrenergic regulation of cardiac myocyte apoptosis. *J Cell Physiol*, 2001; 189(3):257–265.

SUSANTITAPHONG P, CRUZ DN, CERDA J, et al.; Acute Kidney Injury Advisory Group of the American Society of Nephrology. World incidence of AKI: a meta-analysis. *Clin J Am Soc Nephrol*, 2013; 8(9):1482–1493.

THE ACUTE INFARCTION RAMIPRIL EFFICACY (AIRE) STUDY INVESTIGATORS. Effect of ramipril on mortality and morbidity of survivors of acute myocardial infarction with clinical evidence of heart failure. *Lancet*, 1993; 342(8875):821–828.

THE CONSENSUS TRIAL STUDY GROUP. Effects of enalapril on mortality in severe congestive heart failure. *N Engl J Med*, 1987; 316(23):1429–1435.

TOJO A, ONOZATO ML, KOBAYASHI N, et al. Angiotensin II and oxidative stress in Dahl Salt-sensitive rat with heart failure. *Hypertension*, 2002; 40(6):834–839.

TONELLI M, WIEBE N, CULLETON B, et al. Chronic kidney disease and mortality risk: a systematic review. *J Am Soc Nephrol*, 2006; 17(7):2034–2047.

UCHINO S, KELLUM JA, BELLOMO R, et al.; Beginning and Ending Supportive Therapy for the Kidney (BEST Kidney) Investigators. Acute renal failure in critically ill patients: a multinational, multicenter study. *JAMA*, 2005; 294(7):813–818.

VANMASSENHOVE J, KIELSTEIN J, JÖRRES A, BIESEN WV. Management of patients at risk of acute kidney injury. *Lancet*, 2017; 389(10084): 2139–2151.

VAZIRI ND, DICUS M, HO ND, et al. Oxidative stress and dysregulation of superoxide dismutase and NADPH oxidase in renal insufficiency. *Kidney Int*, 2003; 63(1):179–185.

VELAZQUEZ EJ, MORROW DA, DEVORE AD, et al.; PIONEER-HF Investigators. Angiotensin–neprilysin inhibition in acute decompensated heart failure. *N Engl J Med*, Nov 2018; DOI: 10.1056/NEJMoa1812851.

WINTON FR. The influence of venous pressure on the isolated mammalian kidney. *J Physiol*, 1931; 72(1):49–61.

YUSUF S, PITT B, DAVIS CE, et al.; SOLVD Investigators. Effect of enalapril on survival in patients with reduced left ventricular ejection fractions and congestive heart failure. *N Engl J Med*, 1991; 325(5):293–302.

ZANNAD F, MCMURRAY JJ, KRUM H, et al.; EMPHASIS-HF Study Group. Eplerenone in patients with systolic heart failure and mild symptoms. *N Engl J Med*, 2011; 364(1):11–21.

Chapter 2. Overview of the cardiovascular–renal axis in dogs and cats

ACIERNO MJ, BROWN S, COLEMAN AE, et al. ACVIM consensus statement: Guidelines for the identification, evaluation, and management of systemic hypertension in dogs and cats. *J Vet Intern Med*, 2018; 32(6):1803–1822.

HOKAMP JA, NABITY MB. Renal biomarkers in domestic species. *Vet Clin Pathol*, 2016; 45(1):28–56.

MARTINELLI E, LOCATELLI C, BASSIS S, et al. Preliminary investigation of cardiovascular-renal disorders in dogs with chronic mitral valve disease. *J Vet Intern Med*, 2016; 30(5):1612–1618.

ORVALHO JS, COWGILL LD. Cardiorenal syndrome: diagnosis and management. *Vet Clin North Am Small Anim Pract*, 2017; 47(5):1083–1102.

OYAMA MA. Using cardiac biomarkers in veterinary practice. *Vet Clin North Am Small Anim Pract*, 2013; 43(6):1261–1272.

POUCHELON JL, ATKINS CE, BUSSADORI C, et al. Cardiovascular-renal axis disorders in the domestic dog and cat: a veterinary consensus statement. *J Small Anim Pract*, 2015; 56(9):537–552.

RONCO C, HAAPIO M, HOUSE AA, et al. Cardiorenal syndrome. *J Am Coll Cardiol*, 2008; 52(19):1527–1539.

Chapter 3. Renal disorders secondary to cardiovascular disease

Acute cardiovascular disorders causing acute kidney injury

CHOI B-S, MOON H-S, SEO S-H, HYUN C. Evaluation of serum cystatin-C and symmetric dimethylarginine concentrations in dogs with heart failure from chronic mitral valvular insufficiency. *J Vet Med Sci*, 2017; 79(1):41–46.

Martinelli E, Locatelli C, Bassis S, et al. Preliminary investigation of cardiovascular–renal disorders in dogs with chronic mitral valve disease. *J Vet Intern Med*, 2016; 30(5):1612–1618.

Nuñez J, Miñana G, Santas E, Bertomeu-González V. Síndrome cardiorrenal en la insuficiencia cardiaca aguda: revisando paradigmas. *Rev Esp Cardiol*, 2015; 68(5):426–435.

Orvalho JS, Cowgill LD. Cardiorenal syndrome: diagnosis and management. *Vet Clin North Am Small Anim Pract*, 2017; 47(5):1083–1102.

Palazzouoli A, Roucco G. Heart-kidney interactions in cardiorenal syndrome type I. *Adv Chronic Kidney Dis*, 2018; 25(5):408–417.

Ponikowski P, Jankowska EA. Patogenia y presentación clínica de la insuficiencia cardiaca aguda. *Rev Esp Cardiol*, 2015; 68(4):331–337.

Pouchelon JL, Atkins CE, Bussadori C, et al. Cardiovascular-renal axis disorders in the domestic dog and cat: a veterinary consensus statement. *J Small Anim Pract*, 2015; 56(9):537–552.

Rangaswami J, Mathew RO. Pathophysiological mechanisms in cardiorenal syndrome. *Adv Chronic Kidney Dis*, 2018, 25(5):400–407.

Ronco C, Bellasi A, Di Lullo L. Cardiorenal syndrome: an overview. *Adv Chronic Kidney Dis*, 2018; 25(5):382–390.

Ronco C, Cicoira M, McCullough PA. Cardiorenal syndrome type1: pathophysiological crosstalk leading to combined heart and kidney dysfunction in the setting of acutely decompensated heart failure. *J Am Coll Cardiol*, 2012; 60(12):1031–1042.

Chronic cardiovascular disorders leading to chronic kidney disease

Acierno MJ, Brown S, Coleman AE, et al. ACVIM consensus statement: Guidelines for the identification, evaluation, and management of systemic hypertension in dogs and cats. *J Vet Intern Med*, 2018; 32(6):1803–1822.

Atkins CE, Brown WA, Coats JR, et al. Effects of long-term administration of enalapril on clinical indicators of renal function in dogs with compensated mitral regurgitation. *J Am Vet Med Assoc*, 2002; 221(5):654–658.

Boswood A, Murphy A. The effect of heart disease, heart failure and dieresis on selected laboratory and electrocardiographic parameters in dogs. *J Vet Cardiol*, 2006; 8(1):1–9.

Chetboul V, Daste T, Gouni V, et al. Renal resistive index in 55 dogs with degenerative mitral valve disease. *J Vet Intern Med*, 2012; 26(1):101–108.

Choi BS, Moon HS, Seo SH, Hyun C. Evaluation of serum cystatin-C and symmetric dimethylarginine concentrations in dogs with heart failure from chronic mitral valvular insufficiency. *J Vet Med Sci*, 2017; 79(1):41–46.

Gouni V, Chetboul V, Pouchelon JL, et al. Azotemia in cats with feline hypertrophic cardiomyopathy: prevalence and relationships with echocardiographic variables. *J Vet Cardiol*, 2008; 10(2):117–123.

Jung HB, Kang MH, Park HM. Evaluation of serum neutrophil gelatinase-associated lipocalin as a novel biomarker of cardiorenal syndrome in dogs. *J Vet Diagn Invest*, 2018; 30(3):386–391.

Langhorn R, Kieler IN, Koch J, et al. Symmetric dimethylarginine in cats with hypertrophic cardiomyopathy and diabetes mellitus. *J Vet Intern Med*, 2018; 32(1):57–63.

Martinelli E, Locatelli C, Bassis S, et al. Preliminary investigation of cardiovascular–renal disorders in dogs with chronic mitral valve disease. *J Vet Intern Med*, 2016; 30(5):1612–1618.

Nicolle AP, Chetboul V, Allerheiligen T, et al. Azotemia and glomerular filtration rate in dogs with chronic valvular disease. *J Vet Intern Med*, 2007; 21(5):943–949.

Oyama MA. Using cardiac biomarkers in veterinary practice. *Vet Clin North Am Small Anim Pract*, 2013; 43(6):1261–1272.

Pouchelon JL, Atkins CE, Bussadori C, et al. Cardiovascular-renal axis disorders in the domestic dog and cat: a veterinary consensus statement. *J Small Anim Pract*, 2015; 56(9):537–552.

Ronco C, Haapio M, House AA, et al. Cardiorenal syndrome. *J Am Coll Cardiol*, 2008; 52(19):1527–1539.

Savarese A, Probo M, Locatelli C, et al. Reliability of symmetric dimethylarginine in dogs with myxomatous mitral valve disease as kidney biomarker. *Open Vet J*, 2018; 8(3):318–324.

Srivastava M, Ahuja A, Velhankar RD, et al. Cardiorenal syndrome in dilated cardiomyopathy of dogs. *Indian J Can Pract*, 2015; 7(2):94–98.

Vaden SL, Atkins C, Oyama MA. Cardiovascular–renal disorders. In: Elliott J, Grauer GF, Westropp JL (eds.). *BSAVA Manual of Canine and Feline Nephrology and Urology*. Gloucester: British Small Animal Veterinary Association, 2017; pp 196–204.

Yu IB, Huang HP. Prevalence and prognosis of anemia in dogs with degenerative mitral valve disease. *Biomed Res Int*, 2016; 2016:4727054.

Chapter 4. Cardiovascular disorders secondary to kidney disease

Acute kidney disease contributing to impaired cardiac function

Acierno MJ, Labato MA. Kidney diseases and renal replacement therapies. *Vet Clin North Am Small Anim Pract*, 2011; 41.

Clementi A, Virzì GM, Brocca A, et al. Advances in the pathogenesis of cardiorenal syndrome type 3. *Oxid Med Cell Longev*, 2015; Article ID 148082, 8 pages.

Cowgill LD, Guillaumin J. Extracorporeal renal replacement therapy and blood purification in critical care. *J Vet Emerg Crit Care*, 2013; 23(2):194–204.

Di Lullo L, Bellasi A, Barbera V, et al. Pathophysiology of the cardio-renal syndromes types 1–5: An uptodate. *Indian Heart J*, 2017; 69(2):255–265.

Di Lullo L, Bellasi A, Russo D, et al. Cardiorenal acute kidney injury: Epidemiology, presentation, causes, pathophysiology and treatment. *Int J Cardiol*, 2017; 227:143–150.

El-Sherif N, Turitto G. Electrolyte disorders and arrhythmogenesis. *Cardiol J*, 2011; 18(3):233–245.

Keller SP, Kovacevic A, Howard J, et al. Evidence of cardiac injury and arrhythmias in dogs with acute kidney injury. *J Small Anim Pract*, 2016; 57(8):402–408.

Lisciandro GR. Abdominal and thoracic focused assessment with sonography for trauma, triage, and monitoring in small animals. *J Vet Emerg Crit Care (San Antonio)*, 2011; 21(2):104–122.

Orvalho JS, Cowgill LD. Cardiorenal syndrome: diagnosis and management. *Vet Clin North Am Small Anim Pract*, 2017; 47(5):1083–1102.

Pouchelon JL, Atkins CE, Bussadori C, et al. Cardiovascular-renal axis disorders in the domestic dog and cat: a veterinary consensus statement. *J Small Anim Pract*, 2015; 56(9):537–552.

Ronco C, Haapio M, House AA, et al. Cardiorenal syndrome. *J Am Coll Cardiol*, 2008; 52(19):1527–1539.

Schmidt MK, Reynolds CA, Estrada AH, et al. Effect of azotemia on serum N-terminal proBNP concentration in dogs with normal cardiac function: A pilot study. *J Vet Cardiol*, 2009; 11 Suppl 1:S81–S86.

Sharkey LC, Berzina I, Ferasin L, et al. Evaluation of serum cardiac troponin I concentration in dogs with renal failure. *J Am Vet Med Assoc*, 2009; 234(6):767–770.

Yunos NM, Bellomo R, Glassford N, et al. Chloride-liberal vs. chloride-restrictive intravenous fluid administration and acute kidney injury: an extended analysis. *Intensive Care Med*, 2015; 41(2):257–264

Chronic kidney disease contributing to impaired cardiac function

Brown A. Management of chronic kidney disease. In: Elliott J, Grauer G (eds.). *BSAVA Manual of Canine and Feline Nephrology and Urology*. Gloucester (UK): British Small Animal Veterinary Association, 2007; pp. 223–230.

Brown S, Atkins C, Bagley R, et al. Guidelines for the identification, evaluation, and management of systemic hypertension in dogs and cats. *J Vet Intern Med*, 2007; 21(3):542–558.

Brown S. Systemic arterial hypertension. In: Bartges J, Polzin DJ (eds.). *Nephrology and Urology of Small Animals*. Iowa: Wiley-Blackwell, 2011; pp. 676–683.

Buranakarl C, Ankanaporn K, Thammacharoen S, et al. Relationships between degree of azotaemia and blood pressure, urinary protein:creatinine ratio and fractional excretion of electrolytes in dogs with renal azotaemia. *Vet Res Commun*, 2007; 31(3):245–257.

Carlos Sampedrano C, Chetboul V, Gouni V, et al. Systolic and diastolic myocardial dysfunction in cats with hypertrophic cardiomyopathy or systemic hypertension. *J Vet Intern Med*, 2006; 20(5):1106–1115.

Chakrabarti S, Syme HM, Elliott J. Clinicopathological variables predicting progression of azotemia in cats with chronic kidney disease. *J Vet Int Med*, 2012; 26(2):275–281.

Chetboul V, Lefebvre HP, Pinhas C, et al. Spontaneous feline hypertension: clinical and echocardiographic abnormalities, and survival rate. *J Vet Intern Med*, 2003; 17(1):89–95.

Chetboul V, Tissier R. Echocardiographic assessment of canine degenerative mitral valve disease. *J Vet Cardiol*, 2012; 14(1):127–148.

Cheung AK, Sarnak MJ, Yan G, et al. Cardiac diseases in maintenance hemodialysis patients: results of the HEMO Study. *Kidney Int*, 2004; 65(6):2380–2389.

Coleman AE, Brown SA. Hypertension and the kidney. In: Elliott J, Grauer GF, Westropp JL (eds.). *BSAVA Manual of Canine and Feline Nephrology and Urology*. Gloucester: British Small Animal Veterinary Association, 2017; pp. 216–223.

DiBartola SP, de Morais HA. Disorders of potassium: hypokalemia and hyperkalemia. In: DiBartola SP (ed.). *Fluid, Electrolyte, and Acid–Base Disorders in Small Animal Practice*. St. Louis: Saunders Elsevier, 2006; pp. 91–121.

DiBartola SP, Rutgers HC, Zack PM, Tarr MJ. Clinicopathologic findings associated with chronic renal disease in cats: 74 cases (1973–1984). *J Am Vet Med Assoc*, 1987; 190(9):1196–1202.

El Nahas M. Cardio-Kidney-Damage: a unifying concept. *Kidney Int*, 2010; 78(1):14–18.

Elliott J, Barber PJ. Feline chronic renal failure: clinical findings in 80 cases diagnosed between 1992 and 1995. *J Small Anim Pract*, 1998; 39(2):78–85.

Finch N. Measurement of glomerular filtration rate in cats: methods and advantages over routine markers of renal function. *J Feline Med Surg*, 2014; 16(9):736–748.

Finco DR. Association of systemic hypertension with renal injury in dogs with induced renal failure. *J Vet Intern Med*, 2004; 18(3):289–294.

Fonarow GC, Adams KF Jr, Abraham WT, et al. Risk stratification for in-hospital mortality in acutely decompensated heart failure: classification and regression tree analysis. *JAMA*, 2005; 293(5):572–580.

Henik RA, Stepien RL, Bortnowski HB. Spectrum of M-mode echocardiographic abnormalities in 75 cats with systemic hypertension. *J Am Anim Hosp Assoc*, 2004; 40(5):359–363.

Kobayashi DL, Peterson ME, Graves TK, et al. Hypertension in cats with chronic renal failure or hyperthyroidism. *J Vet Int Med*, 1990; 4(2):58–62.

Martínez-Hernández L, Casamian-Sorrosal D, Barrera-Chacón R, et al. Comparison of myocardial damage among dogs at different stages of clinical leishmaniasis and dogs with idiopathic chronic kidney disease. *Vet J*, 2017. 221: 1–5.

Morales DL, Kavarana MN, Helman DN, et al. Restoration of renal function in shock by perfusion of the renal artery with venous blood: a counterintuitive approach. *Crit Care Med*, 2002; 30(6):1297–1300.

O'Neill DG, Elliott J, Church DB, et al. Chronic kidney disease in dogs in UK veterinary practices: prevalence, risk factors, and survival. *J Vet Intern Med*, 2013; 27(4):814–821.

Polzin DJ. Chronic kidney disease. In: Bartges J, Polzin DJ (eds.). *Nephrology and Urology of Small Animals*. Iowa: Wiley-Blackwell, 2011; pp. 433–471.

Pouchelon JL, Atkins CE, Bussadori C, et al. Cardiovascular-renal axis disorders in the domestic dog and cat: a veterinary consensus statement. *J Small Anim Pract*, 2015; 56(9):537–552.

Ronco C, Haapio M, House AA, et al. Cardiorenal syndrome. *J Am Coll Cardiol*, 2008; 52(19):1527–1539.

Segev G. Measurement of blood pressure. In: Elliott J, Grauer GF, Westropp JL (eds.). *BSAVA Manual of Canine and Feline Nephrology and Urology*. Gloucester: British Small Animal Veterinary Association, 2017; pp. 185–194.

Stepien RL. Blood pressure determination. In: Bartges J, Polzin DJ (eds.). *Nephrology and Urology of Small Animals*. Iowa: Wiley-Blackwell, 2011; pp. 86–90.

Sultán MG, Osso JNL. ¿Síndrome cardiorrenal o renocardíaco? Un desafío médico. Parte I. *Insuf Card*, 2006; 1(3) [versión *online*].

Syme H. Hypertension in small animal kidney disease. *Vet Clin North Am Small Anim Pract*, 2011; 41(1):63–89.

Syme HM, Barber PJ, Markwell PJ, Elliott J. Prevalence of systolic hypertension in cats with chronic renal failure at initial evaluation. *J Am Vet Med Assoc*, 2002; 220(12):1799–1804.

Tang WH, Tong W, Jain A, et al. Evaluation and long-term prognosis of new-onset, transient, and persistent anemia in ambulatory patients with chronic heart failure. *J Am Coll Cardiol*, 2008; 51(5):569–576.

Vaden SL, Atkins C, Oyama MA. Cardiovascular–renal disorders. In: Elliott J, Grauer GF, Westropp JL (eds.). *BSAVA Manual of Canine and Feline Nephrology and Urology*. Gloucester: British Small Animal Veterinary Association, 2017; pp. 196–204.

Wilson HE, Jasani S, Wagner TB, et al. Signs of left heart volume overload in severely anaemic cats. *J Feline Med Surg*, 2010; 12(12):904–909.

Chapter 5. Cardiovascular–renal disorders secondary to systemic diseases and concomitant cardiorenal diseases

Acierno MJ, Brown S, Coleman AE, et al. ACVIM consensus statement: Guidelines for the identification, evaluation, and management of systemic hypertension in dogs and cats. *J Vet Intern Med*, 2018; 32(6):1803–1822.

Beier P, Reese S, Holler PJ, et al. The role of hypothyroidism in the etiology and progression of dilated cardiomyopathy in Doberman Pinschers. *J Vet Intern Med*, 2014 Oct 10; 29(1):141–149.

Bond BR, Fox PR, Peterson ME, Skavaril RV. Echocardiographic findings in 103 cats with hyperthyroidism. *J Am Vet Med Assoc*, 1988; 192(11):1546–1549.

Bulmer BJ. Cardiovascular dysfunction in sepsis and critical illness. *Vet Clin North Am Small Anim Pract*, 2011; 41(4):717–726.

Chetboul V, Lefebvre HP, Pinhas C, et al. Spontaneous feline hypertension: clinical and echocardiographic abnormalities, and survival rate. *J Vet Intern Med*, 2003; 17(1):89–95.

Conti-Patara A, de Araújo Caldeira J, de Mattos-Junior E, et al. Changes in tissue perfusion parameters in dogs with severe sepsis/septic shock in response to goal-directed hemodynamic optimization at admission to ICU and the relation to outcome. *J Vet Emerg Crit Care (San Antonio)*, 2012; 22(4):409–418.

Cortadellas O, Del Palacio MJ, Bayón A, et al. Systemic hypertension in dogs with leishmaniasis: prevalence and clinical consequences. *J Vet Intern Med*, 2006; 20(4):941–947.

Dickinson AE, Rozanski EA, Rush JE. Reversible myocardial depression associated with sepsis in a dog. *J Vet Intern Med*, 2007; 21(5):1117–1120.

Diniz PP, de Morais HS, Breitschwerdt EB, Schwartz DS. Serum cardiac troponin I concentration in dogs with ehrlichiosis. *J Vet Intern Med*, 2008; 22(5):1136–1143.

Dutton E, Dukes-McEwan J, Cripps PJ. Serum cardiac troponin I in canine syncope and seizures. *J Vet Cardiol*, 2017; 19(1):1–13.

Fine DM, Tobias AH, Bonagura JD. Cardiovascular manifestations of iatrogenic hyperthyroidism in two dogs. *J Vet Cardiol*, 2010; 12(2):141–146.

Fonfara S, Loureiro J, Swift S, et al. Cardiac troponin I as a marker for severity and prognosis of cardiac disease in dogs. *Vet J*, 2010; 184(3):334–339.

Gow DJ, Gow AG, Bell R, et al. Serum cardiac troponin I in dogs with primary immune-mediated haemolytic anaemia. *J Small Anim Pract*, 2011; 52(5):259–264.

Guglielmini C, Civitella C, Diana A, et al. Serum cardiac troponin I concentration in dogs with precapillary and postcapillary pulmonary hypertension. *J Vet Intern Med*, 2010; 24(1):145–152.

Hamacher L, Dörfelt R, Müller M, Wess G. Serum cardiac troponin I concentrations in dogs with systemic inflammatory response syndrome. *J Vet Intern Med*, 2015; 29(1):164–170.

Keir I, Kellum JA. Acute kidney injury in severe sepsis: pathophysiology, diagnosis, and treatment recommendations. *J Vet Emerg Crit Care (San Antonio)*, 2015; 25(2):200–209.

Kellihan HB, Mackie BA, Stepien RL. NT-proBNP, NT-proANP and cTnI concentrations in dogs with pre-capillary pulmonary hypertension. *J Vet Cardiol*, 2011; 13(3):171–182.

Kenefick S, Parker N, Slater L, Boswood A. Evidence of cardiac autonomic neuropathy in dogs with diabetes mellitus. *Vet Rec*, 2007; 161(3):83–88.

Kim YH, Kim JH, Park C. Evaluation of tissue Doppler ultrasonographic and strain imaging for assessment of myocardial dysfunction in dogs with type 1 diabetes mellitus. *Am J Vet Res*, 2018; 79(10):1035–1043.

Kocaturk M, Martinez S, Eralp O, et al. Tei index (myocardial performance index) and cardiac biomarkers in dogs with parvoviral enteritis. *Res Vet Sci*, 2012; 92(1):24–29.

Lalor SM, Connolly DJ, Elliott J, Syme HM. Plasma concentrations of natriuretic peptides in normal cats and normotensive and hypertensive cats with chronic kidney disease. *J Vet Cardiol*, 2009; 11 Suppl 1:S71–S79.

Langhorn R, Thawley V, Oyama MA, et al. Prediction of long-term outcome by measurement of serum concentration of cardiac troponins in critically ill dogs with systemic inflammation. *J Vet Intern Med*, 2014; 28(5):1492–1497.

Langhorn R, Willesen JL. Cardiac troponins in dogs and cats. *J Vet Intern Med*, 2015 Dec 17; 30(1):36–50.

Little CJ, Gettinby G. Heart failure is common in diabetic cats: findings from a retrospective case-controlled study in first-opinion practice. *J Small Anim Pract*, 2008; 49(1):17–25.

Lobetti R, Dvir E, Pearson J. Cardiac troponins in canine babesiosis. *J Vet Intern Med*, 2002; 16(1):63–68.

Martínez-Hernández L, Casamián-Sorrosal D, Barrera-Chacón R, et al. Comparison of myocardial damage among dogs at different stages of clinical leishmaniasis and dogs with idiopathic chronic kidney disease. *Vet J*, 2017; 221:1–5.

Menaut P, Connolly DJ, Volk A, et al. Circulating natriuretic peptide concentrations in hyperthyroid cats. *J Small Anim Pract*, 2012; 53(12):673–678.

Myers JA, Lunn KF, Bright JM. Echocardiographic findings in 11 cats with acromegaly. *J Vet Intern Med*, 2014; 28(4):1235–1238.

Nelson OL, Thompson PA. Cardiovascular dysfunction in dogs associated with critical illnesses. *J Am Anim Hosp Assoc*, 2006; 42(5):344–349.

Orvalho JS, Cowgill LD. Cardiorenal syndrome: diagnosis and management. *Vet Clin North Am Small Anim Pract*, 2017; 47(5):1083–1102.

Oyama MA, Boswood A, Connolly DJ, et al. Clinical usefulness of an assay for measurement of circulating N-terminal pro-B-type natriuretic peptide concentration in dogs and cats with heart disease. *J Am Vet Med Assoc*, 2013; 243(1):71–82.

Panciera DL. An echocardiographic and electrocardiographic study of cardiovascular function in hypothyroid dogs. *J Am Vet Med Assoc*, 1994; 205(7):996–1000.

Pelander L, Häggström J, Ley CJ, Ljungvall I. Cardiac troponin I and amino-terminal pro B-type natriuretic peptide in dogs with stable chronic kidney disease. *J Vet Intern Med*, 2017; 31(3):805–813.

Pereira NJ, Novo Matos J, Baron Toaldo M, et al. Cats with diabetes mellitus have diastolic dysfunction in the absence of structural heart disease. *Vet J*, 2017; 225:50–55.

Pouchelon JL, Atkins CE, Bussadori C, et al. Cardiovascular-renal axis disorders in the domestic dog and cat: a veterinary consensus statement. *J Small Anim Pract*, 2015; 56(9):537–552.

Raffan E, Loureiro J, Dukes-McEwan J, et al. The cardiac biomarker NT-proBNP is increased in dogs with azotemia. *J Vet Intern Med*, 2009; 23(6):1184–1189.

Ronco C, Haapio M, House AA, et al. Cardiorenal syndrome. *J Am Coll Cardiol*, 2008; 52(19):1527–1539.

Ronco C, House AA, Haapio M. Cardiorenal syndrome: refining the definition of a complex symbiosis gone wrong. *Intensive Care Med*, 2008; 34(5):957–962.

Ronco C, McCullough P, Anker SD, et al. Cardio-renal syndromes: report from the consensus conference of the Acute Dialysis Quality Initiative. *Eur Heart J*, 2009 Dec 25; 31(6):703–711.

Sangster JK, Panciera DL, Abbott JA, *et al.* Cardiac biomarkers in hyperthyroid cats. *J Vet Intern Med*, 2013 Dec 18; 28(2):465–472.

Schober KE, Cornand C, Kirbach B, et al. Serum cardiac troponin I and cardiac troponin T concentrations in dogs with gastric dilatation-volvulus. *J Am Vet Med Assoc*, 2002; 221(3):381–388.

Serra M, Papakonstantinou S, Adamcova M, O'Brien PJ. Veterinary and toxicological applications for the detection of cardiac injury using cardiac troponin. *Vet J*, 2010; 185(1):50–57.

Sharkey LC, Berzina I, Ferasin L, et al. Evaluation of serum cardiac troponin I concentration in dogs with renal failure. *J Am Vet Med Assoc*, 2009; 234(6):767–770.

Syme HM. Cardiovascular and renal manifestations of hyperthyroidism. *Vet Clin North Am Small Anim Pract*, 2007; 37(4):723–743.

Takano H, Kokubu A, Sugimoto K, et al. Left ventricular structural and functional abnormalities in dogs with hyperadrenocorticism. *J Vet Cardiol*, 2015; 17(3):173–181.

Wells SM, Sleeper M. Cardiac troponins. *J Vet Emerg Crit Care*, 2008; 18(3):235–245.

Winter RL, Saunders AB, Gordon SG, *et al.* Biologic variability of N-terminal pro-brain natriuretic peptide in healthy dogs and dogs with myxomatous mitral valve disease. *J Vet Cardiol*, 2017; 19(2):124–131.

Chapter 6. Anaesthetic management of patients with cardiovascular–renal axis disorders

Gowan RA, Baral RM, Lingard AE, et al. A retrospective analysis of the effects of meloxicam on the longevity of aged cats with and without overt chronic kidney disease. *J Feline Med Surg*, 2012; 14(12):876–881.

Holt NE. *Stoelting's Anesthesia and Co-Existing Disease*, 7th ed. Chap. 23: Renal disease. Philadelphia (USA): Elsevier-Health Division, 2017; pp. 425–448.

Martínez-Taboada F, Leece EA. Comparison of propofol with ketofol, a propofol-ketamine admixture, for induction of anaesthesia in healthy dogs. *Vet Anaesth Analg*, 2014; 41(6):575–582.

Meersch M, Schmidt C, Zarbock A. Perioperative acute kidney injury: an under-recognized problem. *Anesth Analg*, 2017; 125(4):1223–1232.

Redondo I. Perianaesthetic mortality in cats: preliminary data of a worldwide multicentric study [poster presentation]. World Congress of Veterinary Anaesthesiologists, Venice, 2018.

Redondo I. Perianaesthetic mortality in dogs: preliminary data of a worldwide multicentric study [poster presentation]. World Congress of Veterinary Anaesthesiologists, Venice, 2018.

Rioja E. Anestesia en pacientes con enfermedad cardiaca (Chapter 1). In: Rioja E, Salazar V, Martínez M, Martínez-Taboada F (eds.). *Manual de anestesia y analgesia de pequeños animales con patologías o condiciones especificas.* Zaragoza (España): Servet editorial, 2016; pp. 1–12.

Rioja E. Anestesia en pacientes con patología renal o urinaria (Chapter 3). In: Rioja E, Salazar V, Martínez M, Martínez-Taboada F (eds.). *Manual de anestesia y analgesia de pequeños animales con patologías o condiciones especificas.* Zaragoza (Spain): Servet editorial, 2016; pp. 27–39.

Rioja E. Urogenital disease (chapter 25). In: *BSAVA Manual of canine and feline anaesthesia and analgesia.* Gloucester (UK): British Small Animal Veterinary Association, 2016; pp. 356–365.

Saporano V, Crovace A, De Marzo L, et al. Echocardiographic evaluation of the cardiovascular effects of medetomidine, acepromazine and their combination in healthy dogs. *Res Vet Sci*, 2013; 95(2):687–692.